Optimizing CBT for PTSD

About the Author

Lily A. Brown, PhD, is a licensed clinical psychologist and Director of the Center for the Treatment and Study of Anxiety at the University of Pennsylvania, Philadelphia, PA. She has published over 100 scientific manuscripts on posttraumatic stress disorder (PTSD), other anxiety-related disorders, and suicide risk. She has received extramural funding from the National Institutes of Health, Department of Defense, and National Science Foundation to support her research.

Optimizing CBT for PTSD

Lily A. Brown

hogrefe

Library of Congress Cataloging in Publication information for the print version of this book is available via the Library of Congress Marc Database under the Library of Congress Control Number 2025947347

Library and Archives Canada Cataloguing in Publication
Title: Optimizing CBT for PTSD / Lily A. Brown.
Names: Brown, Lily A., author.
Description: Includes bibliographical references.
Identifiers: Canadiana (print) 2025027468X | Canadiana (ebook) 20250274701 | ISBN 9780889376694 (softcover) | ISBN 9781613346693 (EPUB) | ISBN 9781616766696 (PDF)
Subjects: LCSH: Cognitive therapy. | LCSH: Post-traumatic stress disorder—Treatment.
Classification: LCC RC489.C63 B76 2025 | DDC 616.89/1425—dc23

www.hogrefe.com

Cover image: © Nice Seven (generated with AI) – Adobe Stock

Publishing Offices
USA: Hogrefe Publishing Corporation, 44 Merrimac St., Newburyport, MA 01950
Phone 978 255 3700; E-mail customersupport@hogrefe.com
EUROPE: Hogrefe Publishing GmbH, Merkelstr. 3, 37085 Göttingen, Germany
Phone +49 551 99950 0, Fax +49 551 99950 111; E-mail publishing@hogrefe.com

Sales & Distribution
USA: Hogrefe Publishing, Customer Services Department, 30 Amberwood Parkway, Ashland, OH 44805
Phone 800 228 3749, Fax 419 281 6883; E-mail customersupport@hogrefe.com
UK: Hogrefe Ltd, Hogrefe House, Albion Place, Oxford, OX1 1QZ
Phone +44 186 579 7920; E-mail customersupport@hogrefe.co.uk
EUROPE: Hogrefe Publishing, Merkelstr. 3, 37085 Göttingen, Germany
Phone +49 551 99950 0, Fax +49 551 99950 111; E-mail publishing@hogrefe.com

Other Offices
CANADA: Hogrefe Publishing Corporation, 82 Laird Drive, East York, Ontario, M4G 3V1
SWITZERLAND: Hogrefe Publishing, Länggass-Strasse 76, 3012 Bern

Printed and bound in the USA

ISBN 978-0-88937-669-4 (print) • ISBN 978-1-61676-669-6 (PDF) • ISBN 978-1-61334-669-3 (EPUB)
https://doi.org/10.1027/00669-000

Contents

1 PTSD Diagnostic Criteria, Prevalence Rates, Comorbidities, and Differential Diagnosis

Diagnostic Criteria

To meet the criteria for posttraumatic stress disorder (PTSD), an individual must report experiencing, witnessing, or learning about a traumatic event. According to the American Psychiatric Association's *Diagnostic and Statistical Manual of Mental Disorders* (5th ed., text rev.; DSM-5-TR) (2022), traumatic events include (but are not limited to) threats to one's physical integrity, such as physical or sexual assault, natural disasters, life-threatening illness or injury, serious accidents, or combat exposure. DSM-5-TR also considers occupational exposure to trauma or repeated exposure to the details of others' trauma as grounds for a criterion A trauma. As will become clear later, exposure to a trauma alone is insufficient for a diagnosis of PTSD; trauma exposure must be accompanied by symptoms from the following clusters: intrusions (criterion B; 1 symptom); avoidance (criterion C; 1 symptom); negative alterations in cognitions or mood (criterion D; 2 symptoms); and alterations in arousal and reactivity (criterion E; 2 symptoms). Symptoms must last at least one month (criterion F) and cause clinically significant distress or impairment (criterion G). Finally, the symptoms cannot be purely substance-induced or attributable to a medical condition. Some individuals experience dissociative symptoms that accompany PTSD, which are either of a depersonalized (feelings of detachment) or derealized (experiences of unreality) nature.

Prevalence

The most commonly experienced traumatic events in the United States include exposure to physical or sexual assault, with over 53% of women and 29% of men reporting sexual violence (Basile et al., 2022) and witnessing such assaults (Coalition for National Trauma Research, 2024). The unexpected death of a loved one affects over 50% of US adults (Benjet et al., 2016), while natural disasters affect approximately 19–25% of Americans, especially those living in disaster-prone areas (Kessler et al., 2017). Serious accidents, such as motor vehicle crashes, fires, or severe injuries, are reported by 25–35% of individuals, highlighting the widespread nature of such traumatic experiences (Coalition for National Trauma Research, 2024).

Most people will directly experience, witness, or learn about a traumatic event (Kilpatrick et al., 2013) at some point in their life. The traumatic events experienced most frequently in the United States include exposure to physical or sexual assault (53%), death of a family member/close friend due to violence/disaster (51.8%), disaster (50.5%), or accident/fire (48.3), and witnessing physical or sexual assault (33.2%) (Kilpatrick et al., 2013). Survivors of interpersonal trauma and combat have the highest rates of PTSD (Reger et al., 2019). Fortunately, despite the near-ubiquitous exposure to trauma, lifetime rates of PTSD are between 8–9%, with rates among people who identify as women (12.8%) twice as high as those among people who identify as men (5.7%; Kilpatrick et al., 2013). Gender differences in the rate of PTSD may partially be explained by the type of trauma to which people are exposed, as when people with the same index trauma type are studied (i.e., motor vehicle accident), rates of PTSD diagnosis are similar, though still somewhat higher among women (Olff, 2017).

Individuals who identify as a member of the lesbian, gay, bisexual, transgender, and queer/questioning (LGBTQ+) community report significantly higher rates of exposure to trauma compared to the general population (Craig et al., 2020). In terms of race, Black and Latina/Latino individuals are more likely to meet criteria for PTSD than White individuals but often report lower overall PTSD severity (Ruglass et al., 2020). Approximately 38–45% of patients with PTSD meet criteria for the dissociative subtype (Swart et al., 2020; White et al., 2022). About one in four patients (24.8%) report delayed symptoms of PTSD (Utzon-Frank et al., 2014), but most of those who experience delayed PTSD report elevated subthreshold symptoms in the immediate aftermath of the traumatic event compared to patients who never meet criteria for PTSD (Bonde et al., 2022).

Comorbidities

Psychiatric Comorbidities

PTSD has very high rates of comorbidity with other psychiatric illnesses, with some estimates as high at 90% of patients with PTSD who meet criteria for a secondary disorder (Roberts et al., 2020). Comorbidity between PTSD and anxiety disorders is high, with 28% of patients with PTSD meeting criteria for generalized anxiety disorder, 24% for panic disorder with/without agoraphobia, 1% for agoraphobia, 19% for social anxiety disorder, and 37% for specific phobia (Pietrzak et al., 2011).

PTSD is highly comorbid with substance use disorders, with 36–52% meeting criteria for alcohol use disorder, 46–66% for substance use disorder, 40–60% for nicotine use disorder, and 46% for any substance use disorder (Houghton et al., 2023) A systematic review (Hawn et al., 2020) provided some evidence supporting a self-medication hypothesis between PTSD and substance use, although the authors noted some significant challenges with methodological rigor of the studies available for inclusion (particularly related to the measurement of trauma-related drinking to cope). The relationship between PTSD and alcohol use problems is mediated by trauma-related drinking to cope (Hawn et al., 2020), and therefore, it is essential to assess substance use in patients with PTSD prior to beginning cognitive behavioral therapy (CBT) for PTSD.

In network analyses in which the central symptoms of PTSD were explored separately from, and then in combination with, depression symptoms, intrusion symptoms were central to PTSD alone, and concentration difficulties and anhedonia were central to the combined network (Duek et al., 2021), suggesting that these two symptoms help explain the high rates of comorbidity between depression and PTSD. Approximately 35% of patients with PTSD also meet criteria for major depressive disorder, 10% for dysthymic disorder/persistent depressive disorder, 19% for bipolar I disorder, and 4% for bipolar II disorder, with 61.5% meeting criteria for any mood disorder (Pietrzak et al., 2011). Depression and PTSD symptoms are so intimately linked that improvements in one condition in CBT for PTSD predicts improvements in the other condition, and vice versa (Brown, Jerud, et al., 2018).

Approximately 14% of patients with PTSD report a lifetime history of suicide attempts (Pietrzak et al., 2011), and PTSD increases the risk of death by suicide nearly tenfold (Gradus et al., 2010; Pompili et al., 2013). Most trauma types are associated with higher rates of suicidal ideation and attempt risk among individuals with PTSD compared to those without PTSD (for details on managing suicide risk, see Chapter 10), and individuals with a history of childhood maltreatment and assault have some of the highest rates of suicidal ideation (approximately 50%; LeBouthillier et al., 2015). Furthermore, some individuals who survive a suicide attempt can develop PTSD from the attempt itself, although this is an underresearched topic (Stanley, Boffa, et al., 2019; Stanley, Hom, et al., 2019).

Myriad other psychiatric illnesses are also experienced at higher rates among patients with PTSD, including eating disorders (Brewerton et al., 2020; Scharff et al., 2021), traumatic brain injury (Rosen & Ayers, 2020), borderline personality disorder (Ford & Courtois, 2021), and sleep disorders (Elliott et al., 2020; Roberts et al., 2020). Comorbidity is the norm rather than the exception, and clinicians who are preparing to deliver CBT for PTSD must anticipate that their patients will also have comorbid symptoms that occasionally require attention. Fortunately, meta-analyses have largely revealed that comorbid conditions improve after getting CBT for PTSD, specifically prolonged exposure (PE) therapy (van Minnen et al., 2015).

Medical Comorbidities

In addition to psychiatric comorbidities, there are a variety of medical comorbidities that are more likely among patients with PTSD. These include metabolic syndrome (Rosenbaum et al., 2015; Weiss et al., 2011), cardiovascular disease (Edmondson & Känel, 2017; O'Donnell et al., 2021), pain (Kind & Otis, 2019), and gastrointestinal illness (Pacella et al., 2013). Patients who receive CBT for PTSD (specifically PE) experience improvement in physical health over time (Rauch et al., 2009). In addition, patients who receive PE have less overutilization of medical services following treatment (Tuerk et al., 2013). Therefore, it is essential that patients with PTSD are referred for evidence-based treatments for PTSD; and CBT has the strongest evidence base to date (American Psychological Association, 2017; VA/DoD, 2023).

Evidence-Based Assessments for PTSD

Clinical practice guidelines (VA/DoD, 2023) recommend the Primary Care PTSD Screen for DSM-5 (PC-PTSD-5; Prins et al., 2016) for screening for PTSD, the Clinician-Administered PTSD Scale for DSM-5 (CAPS-5; Weathers et al., 2018) or the Posttraumatic Stress Disorder Symptom Scale – Interview for DSM-5 (PSSI-5; Foa, McLean, Zang, Zhong, Rauch, et al., 2016) for confirming a PTSD diagnosis, and the PTSD Checklist for DSM-5 (Bovin et al., 2016) for monitoring changes in symptoms over time. Another commonly used self-report assessment is the Posttraumatic Diagnostic Scale for DSM-5 (PDS-5; Foa, McLean, Zang, Zhong, Powers, et al., 2016). However, the evidence supporting each of these recommended screeners/assessments is "weak" according to guideline standards, meaning that more work needs to be done to establish the optimal assessment options.

Evidence-Based Treatments for PTSD

Clinical practice guidelines (American Psychological Association, 2017; VA/DoD, 2023) strongly recommend psychotherapy for PTSD over pharmacologic intervention, and the therapies with the strongest recommendations include cognitive processing therapy (CPT) and PE (both types of CBT) and eye-movement desensitization and reprocessing (EMDR). Additional psychotherapies that are recommended (with weak support, but this may increase over time) include Ehlers' cognitive therapy for PTSD (Ehlers et al., 2005), written exposure therapy (Sloan & Marx, 2019), and present-centered therapy (Schnurr et al., 2003). There is a long list of additional therapies that purport to treat PTSD but are currently not recommended. In summary, CBT for PTSD has the strongest evidence base, and in this book, I will describe cognitive and behavioral interventions to target PTSD symptoms directly.

Cultural Considerations

As with all CBT, a patient's cultural context affects many aspects of their assessment and treatment for PTSD. For instance, some patients will benefit from a more unstructured introductory assessment to build rapport and comfort prior to transitioning into a formal structured clinical assessment. In contrast, other patients might strongly prefer a structured diagnostic assessment because the clinical encounter will resemble other healthcare encounters. Likewise, some patients may benefit from additional preparatory sessions prior to officially beginning CBT for PTSD to build comfort, whereas other patients might prefer to dive into the content immediately. It is essential to gain a certain understanding of the patient's culture and expectations for assessment and therapy to best offer them the service that they desire and benefit from when offering CBT for PTSD.

In this context, clinicians further benefit from some understanding of the patient's culture, but also about how the patient's worldview differs from their own. As discussed in detail in Chapter 9, traumas can fundamentally alter the ways that individuals view themselves, other people, and the world. For instance, a patient who grew up in a collectivistic culture might begin to shift their priorities after exposure to a trauma if they perceive that other people cannot be trusted. Conversely, a patient who grew up in a highly individualized culture might start to doubt their own abilities following a trauma and begin to rely more heavily on a support network due to lowered self-esteem. Thus, it is essential to gain an understanding of the patient's self-description of the culture in which they were raised, but also to assess how their viewpoints differ from their culture of origin.

The delivery of CBT for PTSD also varies as a function of the patient's age, and this book was written with an emphasis on the treatment of PTSD in adults. Most of the techniques described in this book have relevance across the lifespan, and I briefly describe lifespan adaptations as relevant. However, some techniques are more successful for younger patients when parental support is enlisted, and some techniques might not be fruitful if a patient is too young, even with parental support. In such cases, following a trauma-focused CBT protocol is recommended (Cohen et al., 2006).

Summary

In this chapter, I discussed diagnostic features of PTSD as well as the prevalence of exposure to different types of traumatic events. In addition, I outlined prevalence rates of PTSD as well as details about psychiatric and medical comorbidities. I discussed a broad overview of the evidence-based data connected to CBT for PTSD, based on clinical practice guidelines, and conclude with some coverage of cultural considerations.

2 Maintenance of Distress in PTSD

CBT for PTSD focuses on addressing the cognitions and behaviors that maintain PTSD over time. In this chapter, I review the evidence for cognitive and behavioral factors that contribute to maintenance or exacerbation of PTSD, as these are the focus of CBT in the remainder of this book. Understanding the contributors to the development and maintenance of PTSD symptoms forms the basis of understanding the rationale behind the decisions that therapists make to conceptualize and deliver interventions in CBT for PTSD.

Cognitive Contributors to the Maintenance of PTSD

As discussed in Chapter 1, changes in cognitions about the self, the world, or other people are now reflected in the symptom criteria for PTSD. Prior to this diagnostic consideration, trauma-related cognitions related to mental defeat, confusion about the trauma, negative appraisals of emotional reactions to the trauma, negative appraisals of PTSD symptoms, negative perceptions of how others responded to the trauma, and the perception that life is permanently changed by the trauma were each associated with both the onset and maintenance of PTSD (Dunmore et al., 1999). These types of trauma-related cognitions are formally assessed in the Posttraumatic Cognitions Inventory (PTCI; Foa et al., 1999), which I recommend that clinicians incorporate into their treatment planning for patients receiving CBT for PTSD (see also Chapter 9). A briefer version, the PTCI-9, has some psychometric validation as well (Wells et al., 2019).

Some research supports the finding that the perception of threat to life during the trauma is associated with the development and maintenance of PTSD (Meiser-Stedman et al., 2019; Schnurr et al., 2004), whereas other studies found that perceptions of danger during the trauma did not predict the development or maintenance of PTSD (Beck et al., 2006). This might partially depend on the nature of the index trauma, given that some index traumas are catastrophic for patients even if they do not perceive a risk of imminent death. For instance, a patient who is being raped might not think that the rapist will murder her but nonetheless might experience severe symptoms of PTSD in the aftermath of the trauma.

Following exposure to a trauma, patients who do not *perceive* positive responses from others are more likely to meet criteria for PTSD (Simon et al., 2019). When someone in the support network attempts to convey sympathy but a trauma survivor interprets this reaction as an indication that they are weak, this can be associated with the onset of PTSD. Difficulties with connecting to others is a hallmark feature of PTSD that might be exacerbated by cognitive shifts and interpretations of how people in the support network are responding to the patient.

My colleagues and I published a review of the role of negative cognitions about oneself, others, and the world, in which we demonstrated that these cognitions are key to response to CBT treatment (Brown et al., 2019). Improvement in trauma-related cognitions in CBT for PTSD predicted improvement in PTSD symptoms (Brown et al., 2019). However, these results were confounded by the fact that DSM-5 symptoms include trauma-related cognitions, so there is some overlap in these variables in more recent studies. Nevertheless, prior to the DSM-5 findings, there were consistent reports covered in the review suggesting that changes in trauma-related cognitions are essential to improve PTSD symptoms in CBT for PTSD. For these reasons, CBT for PTSD always includes some focus on addressing trauma-related cognitions, although the manner of addressing cognitions might differ based on the approach being used. More details on addressing trauma-related cognitions in CBT for PTSD are covered in Chapter 9.

Avoidance

Avoidance is a hallmark feature of PTSD and a core treatment target in CBT for PTSD. Avoidant coping shortly after exposure to a trauma is a strong predictor of PTSD symptoms in the future (Difede & Barocas, 1999; Krause et al., 2008; Pineles et al., 2011). Emotional avoidance also predicts comorbid symptoms of PTSD, including depression (Forbes et al., 2020). Avoidance is so pervasive among patients with PTSD that it persists even when it costs them important benefits or rewards (Weaver et al., 2020). Psychological detachment during the trauma itself (a form of dissociation) predicts the onset of PTSD (Dunmore et al., 1999; Meiser-Stedman et al., 2019; Schnurr et al., 2004).

Patients who engage in a ruminative style of thinking about the trauma with a goal of "undoing" the negative consequences are also more likely to develop PTSD (Dunmore et al., 1999). Rumination about the trauma is especially predictive of PTSD when the rumination lacks concrete details about the trauma and is more abstract in nature (Ehring et al., 2008). This rumination behavior can serve the function of avoidance because for some patients with PTSD, ruminating about the trauma offers a chance to try to "figure it out" and prevent something similar happening again.

Patients who report higher rates of avoidance as a coping strategy at the beginning of treatment for PTSD (across a range of therapies) report higher PTSD severity at the end of treatment (Badour et al., 2012). This is why a primary target of CBT for PTSD is teaching patients to approach rather than avoid as a primary way of coping with anxiety. As discussed in Chapter 3, exposure therapy practices are a primary strategy for directly addressing and reducing avoidance.

Additional Contributors to the Onset and Maintenance of PTSD

Some additional factors are associated with the onset or maintenance of PTSD that are not covered under the larger umbrella of trauma-related cognitions or avoidance. In one study of veterans, a variety of demographic and psychosocial factors were associated with PTSD, including lower socioeconomic status before military enlistment, emotional support upon homecoming, and additional trauma exposure following military discharge (in addition to dissociation during the trauma and perception of life threat, as mentioned previously; Schnurr et al., 2004). In civilian survivors of motor vehicle accidents, pretrauma unemployment predicted the development of PTSD, and this effect was especially strong among individuals who identified as men (Beck et al., 2006); social support predicts improvement in PTSD symptoms among patients in this population who initially report PTSD symptoms in the first month after a trauma (Robinaugh et al., 2011). As might be obvious, demographic factors such as employment and income are not easily modifiable in therapy and are not usually a focus of CBT for PTSD. However, in some cases, PTSD symptoms can interfere with school and occupational attainment and treatment can help improve occupational outcomes. Social support is not typically a direct target of CBT for PTSD, but we do often include a family-based psychoeducation session as appropriate to elicit additional social support (see Chapter 15), and behavioral activation can be used to improve social connections (see Chapter 8). Thus, while avoidance and trauma-related cognitions are core targets of CBT for PTSD, there are numerous opportunities for targeting other factors that are correlated with PTSD-related distress.

Summary

In this chapter, I discussed some of the factors that are known to contribute to the development and maintenance of PTSD. In particular, I covered trauma-related cognitions and avoidance as core features that contribute to symptom onset, maintenance, and exacerbation. Finally, I reviewed some of the research on demographic factors that are associated with the onset of PTSD as well as with treatment response.

3 Exposure Therapy: Findings From the Laboratory

Exposure therapy has its origins in experimental manipulations of fear conditioning and extinction training. Given that much of what we know about exposure therapy comes directly from findings in the laboratory, in this chapter, I briefly review experimental principles relevant to exposure therapy. By understanding these principles, it is possible to think conceptually about strategies to improve the potential for extinction learning in CBT for PTSD to help you and your patient get unstuck from difficult moments in therapy.

A Few Notes About Experimental Analogs for PTSD

Some PTSD experts in the field feel strongly that experimental analogs of fear conditioning and extinction are woefully inadequate for understanding PTSD in humans. These skeptics raise valid points for consideration of which all CBT therapists should be aware. First, fear conditioning may be an inadequate explanation for understanding the impact of a trauma. Indeed, traumas have an emotional impact that extends far beyond fear and includes shame, guilt, and moral injury, to name just a few. Fortunately, even though exposure therapy began as a strategy to address fear, it now has evidence for improving comorbid emotions, such as guilt and shame (Kubany & Ralston, 2006; McLean et al., 2019). Second, extinction training alone might be insufficient to deal with the complex needs that a survivor of trauma must address in therapy. This is a valid criticism, given that exposure therapy does not *directly* address trauma-related cognitions in the manner that other CBT strategies do (i.e., cognitive restructuring), and given that not all patients benefit from exposure therapy (response rates range from 19% to 63%, depending on the study; Bilek et al., 2022; Roth-Rawald et al., 2023). However, exposure therapy has some of the strongest evidence of all therapies for PTSD (Cusack et al., 2016). While it is not a panacea, it can work wonders for a large proportion of patients with PTSD, with 66% more patients achieving remission from PTSD if they receive exposure therapy compared to those on a waiting list (rates for other treatments versus untreated controls: 50% for cognitive therapy; 44% for cognitive processing therapy (CPT) specifically; and 26% for mixed CBT; Cusack et al., 2016). Thus, fear conditioning and extinction models might be insufficient for understanding some of the clinical complexities of working with patients with PTSD. However, these laboratory models provide useful insights into phenomena that are reliably observed in clinical presentations of PTSD, and for that reason, they should be understood to help improve clinical decision-making when delivering exposure therapy as part of CBT for PTSD.

Fear Conditioning

In experimental studies of fear conditioning, a benign, nonbiologically significant stimulus (conditioned stimulus; CS) is presented in combination with a biologically significant stimulus (unconditioned stimulus; US). This pairing between a significant and insignificant stimulus results in learning about the insignificant stimulus in a process called "conditioning." In human studies of fear conditioning, the CS is usually a neutral sound or an image and is often presented to the participant for several seconds before the US, which is usually an aversive muscle stimulation (i.e., electric shock) or in some cases an aversive loud noise. The CS and US typically coterminate (i.e., end together). The participant will typically go through an experimental design where the CS is presented multiple times, and 75% of the time, it will be reinforced with the aversive US (a 75% reinforcement ratio). In some studies, one CS, CS_A, is paired with a US and the other, CS_B, is not. This design allows the experimenter to compare different rates of responding to each CS to learn about fear and safety learning. The rate of fear conditioning is measured in terms of the conditioned response (CR), which could be a subjective response, such as subjective units of distress or expectancy of the US; a physiological response, such as skin conductance response or heart rate; or a neurological response, such as blood oxygenation level-dependent response in a functional magnetic resonance imaging scanner.

In extinction training, the CS is presented in the absence of the US. In experimental designs where there are multiple CS types (i.e., CS_A and CS_B), they might both be presented during extinction training. Sometimes experimenters will divide extinction training into early (e.g., the first 2–4 trials), middle (e.g., the next 2–4 trials) and late extinction training (e.g., the last 2–4 trials) based on the number of extinction trials that a participant completes in a round of extinction training to evaluate differences in the rate of the CR (extinction learning expression) or the mean CR over time during these windows. An experimenter might have one or more rounds of trials for extinction retention.

Table 1. Types of return of fear, their definition, and their clinical management in exposure therapy

Type of return of fear	Definition and example in the laboratory	Clinical example	Clinical management
Spontaneous recovery	Return of fear due to the passage of time alone; a subject has little CR at the end of extinction training, but after the passage of time, when tested for extinction retention with a presentation of the CS, the CR returns.	The patient is doing well in exposure therapy and is reporting low rates of fear and anxiety after several sessions. Then, the patient takes a break from exposure therapy for a few weeks and when they return, their fear is increased again.	Remind the patient to continue exposure therapy practice between sessions, including when they are on breaks from therapy or when they are tapering the frequency of sessions. Provide psychoeducation that return of fear after the passage of time is very normal and should not be a source of concern. If they continue practicing exposure therapy, they are likely to resolve the issue quickly (relative to the amount of time that learning initially took in therapy). The more that they can continue practicing exposures between sessions and after therapy is completed, the less likely it is that spontaneous recovery will set them back in their progress.
Rapid reacquisition	Return of fear following extinction training.When the CS is paired with the US for a reinforced trial, the CR will return.	A patient with PTSD from a motor vehicle accident is doing well in exposure therapy and has a reduction in fear and anxiety associated with driving. Then, the patient has another car accident. Fear and anxiety about driving return.	Provide psychoeducation to the patient about rapid reacquisition. Tell the patient that while we only do exposures that we collectively deem as objectively safe, there is no way to guarantee the patient's complete safety. There is still a chance that they could get into a car accident when doing exposure therapy practice or in other situations. Remind them that if this happens, it is likely that they will experience a surge in their fear and anxiety. Provide them with psychoeducation that if they continue with exposure practice after this stressful experience, exposure therapy can work just as effectively next time. For some patients, the next exposure therapy will reduce their fear even more quickly compared to the first time that they went through the exposure.

continued on next page

Table 1. Continued

Type of return of fear	Definition and example in the laboratory	Clinical example	Clinical management
Reinstatement	Return of fear following extinction training with an unpaired US presentation (i.e., a US presented without a CS).	The patient is doing well in exposure therapy and suddenly experiences a very stressful (or even another traumatic) event. Fear to the CS related to the original trauma returns.	Provide psychoeducation about the possibility that reinstatement can happen. Specifically, educate patients that as they experience new, stressful events, they may notice that their distress about their trauma may return. It can be helpful to tell them that the research on reinstatement is less clear than on some other types of return of fear (i.e., renewal and spontaneous recovery), but it can be helpful to know about how it might emerge.
Renewal	Return of fear following extinction training when the CS is presented in a novel context.	The patient is doing well to exposures that they practice in your therapy office, but when they attempt to do the practices at home, their distress is very high.	Practice exposure in as many settings as possible, including in the therapy office, at the patient's home, and in the general community wherever possible. Also consider varying the internal context for the participant, including their level of fatigue prior to an exposure, whether they have had coffee or another stimulant and whether they feel like doing the exposure. Educate the patient that variation in the locations and physical states will help them maintain their gains. Some patients might know about the concept of state-dependent learning; that is, what we learn in one state will be recalled more easily when we are in that state again.

Finally, tests of extinction retention involve an evaluation of CR after some delay following extinction training, which could be a day, a week, or longer, depending on the research question. Tests of extinction retention aim to evaluate the extent to which learning that occurred during extinction training is retained later. These tests can sometimes include experimental manipulations to evaluate the return of fear in the form of spontaneous recovery, reinstatement, rapid reacquisition, and renewal, each described next (and in Table 1).

Often, extinction retention tests will include a few trials of the CS without the US. When the CR is higher at the beginning of extinction retention tests compared to at the end of extinction training, this can serve as evidence of spontaneous recovery, which is a return of the CR in response to the CS following extinction training due to the passage of time alone. In some experiments, the experimenter may include a test of reinstatement, in which an unpaired US presentation occurs (typically on an intertrial interval, which is the time between CS presentations) to evaluate changes in the CR during the next presentation of the CS. In other experiments, extinction retention will include an occasional CS–US pairing to evaluate the CR on the next unpaired trial of the CS and evaluate the rate of reacquisition of fear conditioning. Finally, some experiments will evaluate tests of renewal of the CR, during which the context of testing is different from the context of extinction training and the experimenter evaluates the impact of these context changes on the level of the CR in response to a presentation of the CS.

Parallels Between Fear Conditioning and Trauma Exposure

When a patient is exposed to trauma, there are numerous internal and external cues that can become paired with a perception of danger, in a process that mirrors fear conditioning. The trauma itself is a biologically significant US. The CS can include features of the context or the assailant, internal experiences or thoughts, and objects or cues that were present during the trauma. Note that it can be helpful to become aware of examples of CS types because these can become the foundation of *in vivo* exposure practice in CBT for PTSD (see Chapter 5). Contextual cues include the city or state or country where a trauma occurred; whether the trauma occurred in an urban, suburban, or rural area; the type of street where the trauma occurred; the type of location in general where the trauma occurred; the colors on the walls or other materials relevant to the room in which the trauma occurred; the time of day for the trauma; how densely or sparsely populated an area was during the trauma; the level of noise outside during the trauma; and the temperature, to name just a few. For example, my father was a veteran of the Vietnam War, and he was drafted to serve in the Army infantry in 1968–1969 as a gunner's assistant, and later (when his gunner was killed in action), as a gunner. He witnessed unthinkable traumas that he never disclosed to our family before his death in 2016, but he was open about how the war affected him his entire life. When I had my first apartment in college, he came to visit during the hot summer months. He put one foot inside the apartment, immediately said, "It feels like Vietnam in here – [expletive] this," and we immediately went to buy a window air conditioner. It was an eye-opener to me that the war was with him wherever he was.

Features of the assailant can include all their physical features, such as eye color, skin color, body build, hair type, height, distinct facial or bodily features, and the clothes that the assailant was wearing. Internal experiences can include emotions, physical sensations, and thoughts that the trauma survivor experienced during the trauma. Other objects or cues that are in the surrounding area during the trauma can also become part of the package of CS, including holsters for weapons (the weapons themselves might be USs depending on the patient's interpretation of the weapon before a trauma); objects that are not typically weapons but that were used as weapons against a survivor, such as keys, plastic bags, cords, or others; and objects that were not directly related to the trauma but that serve as a reminder of the trauma, such as music or media that were in the background; sheets on a bed or decorations in a room; the scent of a notable cologne or perfume worn by an assailant of a trauma; the type of or paint on a car that was involved in a trauma; and jewelry or clothes that the survivor was wearing during the trauma. Each of these internal or external cues can become paired with the perception of danger or reminders of the trauma and become sources of avoidance for a survivor with PTSD.

Parallels Between Extinction Training, Extinction Retention, and Exposure Therapy

As with extinction training, exposure therapy involves the confronting of stimuli that a survivor with PTSD is avoiding following exposure to a trauma in the absence of a US. As discussed in the full discussion of *in vivo* exposure in Chapter 5, the goal during *in vivo* exposure sessions is to coach a patient to repeatedly approach objects, situations, or people that remind them of the trauma, and to do so while tracking whether the patient's fears about the exposure came to fruition (i.e., whether expectation violation occurred).

Therapists should design exposures in a manner that allows them to anticipate and prevent future return of fear. That involves varying the amount of time between exposure sessions to allow for spontaneous recovery to occur, and then giving the patient an opportunity to push through their return of fear and feel accomplished in doing so. It also involves helping patients to continue exposure practice even if they have had occasional reinforced trials in which a negative outcome (US) occurs during exposure, and helping patients to highlight how they got through that difficult situation, and, most importantly, how they continue with exposure practice later. In addition, patients who experience unrelated stressful events might experience a return of fear, like reinstatement, and would benefit from proactive brainstorming around how to stay on track even in this case.

Varying the context of exposure therapy practice is essential, given that extinction learning is context-dependent but often fear conditioning is not. Thus, exposure sessions must occur outside the traditional therapeutic setting. It can be helpful to remind participants that exposure therapy will be most successful when they have an opportunity to practice exposures in a variety of locations and with a variety of circumstances to promote long-term retention of learning. Contextual variation also includes alterations to the *internal* context for a patient, which can include altering their body temperature, caffeine consumption, and energy level prior to an exposure to achieve optimal retention of learning.

Summary

In this chapter, I described fear conditioning and extinction as an experimental analog to exposure therapy in the context of CBT for PTSD. I reviewed four indicators of return of fear—namely, spontaneous recovery, rapid reacquisition, reinstatement, and renewal. Then I discussed some strategies to manage return of fear clinically in order to optimize response rates from exposure therapy in CBT for PTSD.

4 Psychoeducation and Getting Buy-in for CBT for PTSD

In providing consultation to many therapists who are new to CBT for PTSD, I have learned that the manner in which a therapist provides their "pitch" for a treatment has a major impact on whether a patient ultimately agrees to the treatment plan. Ideally, therapists can balance flexibility in their pitch for why a particular therapeutic approach was selected with the confidence that they are guiding their decisions by the research literature. Therapists should also balance patient preference for a particular theoretical orientation against their own limitations in their expertise in certain approaches. For instance, in my center, the Center for the Treatment and Study of Anxiety at the University of Pennsylvania, patients exclusively receive CBT. This means that buy-in around the treatment plan begins from the point where patients visit our website, continues during the initial screening process, and is deepened during the initial intake evaluation. In facilities that offer multiple therapeutic approaches for PTSD, therapists need to be familiar with how to discuss CBT with patients in a way that is palatable and acceptable.

The Rationale for CBT in General

The rationale for CBT for PTSD highlights several fundamental principles that are relevant to CBT for any condition, as well as treatment features that are unique to the experience of PTSD. The general rationale for CBT is focused on the cognitive model, which I describe in detail in several of the subsequent chapters of this book and which comes from cognitive therapy (Beck, 2010). According to this model, every emotion is comprised of three core components: cognitions, behaviors/behavioral urges, and physical sensations. Each of these three components contributes to the others in increasing or decreasing the intensity of a given emotion. Here, I describe a general strategy for describing the cognitive model to a patient with PTSD.

Therapist: If it's okay with you, I would like to explain a bit about why we approach therapy as we do in CBT. Would it be acceptable to you if we took some time to discuss this?

Patient: Yes, I would like to understand it better.

Therapist: Great. The basic idea is that every emotion has three important parts to it. The first one is the cognitive or thinking part. The cognitive part is whatever thoughts go through your mind when you feel a particular emotion that makes that emotion make sense to you. The second part is the behavior or behavior urge part, which is what you do or are tempted to do when you feel an emotion. Usually, those behaviors are the things that you're tempted to do to try to help yourself feel better in the moment, whether or not they work in the long run. The third part is the physical sensation—that's what you feel in your body when you experience a given emotion. Does this make sense so far?

Patient: I guess so—I just know that when I feel emotions, they hit me quickly and I get flustered quickly, and sometimes don't know what to do. It's like my animal instincts kick in and sometimes I do things I regret.

Therapist: That's a really good analogy, and what you just described is a really common experience. The goal of this therapy is helping you to slow down your emotions a bit and to understand them better so that you can respond differently the next time you have them. It's also about learning strategies in advance to know what to do to decrease the intensity of difficult emotions where possible. How does that sound to you?

Patient: That's what I'm here for—my PTSD has been harassing me for so long that I feel like I'm out of control sometimes.

Therapist: Yes, a key goal of this therapy is helping you to increase your sense of control. So, in addition to each emotion having these three parts, each of the parts tends to amplify the others. What you're thinking in a situation affects how you physically feel, which affects what you think you can or should do, which further affects how you feel and what you think. Each of the parts is closely connected to the others—we call this the "cognitive model." It helps to explain why sometimes our emotions can spiral so quickly and why people can feel like their emotions are out of their control. In CBT, the goal is to help you realize the control that you have.

Patient: OK, but I'm sure that realizing this about my emotions isn't going to change much about them.

Therapist: I agree with you, so we'll take it a step further. In CBT, we can work on each of the emotional components separately to help you learn skills for how to manage your emotions differently. Some of the skills that we're going to work on will be behavioral skills, whereas some will be cognitive skills and some might be skills to respond differently to physical sensations. Each patient is unique, and so the emphasis that we place on each of these domains varies based on your needs. You and I will come up with a treatment plan together to help you to slow down your emotions, understand them better, and respond differently to them.

To summarize, the goal of the general rationale for CBT for any condition is highlighting that every emotion has distinct, discernable components. By understanding these components with greater clarity, patients will gain an opportunity to respond to emotions differently to reduce the intensity of the emotions in the future.

The Rationale for CBT for PTSD

The rationale for CBT for PTSD centers around two core components that are known to contribute to the development and maintenance of PTSD: avoidance and trauma-related cognitions. Below, I describe a rationale for treatment that highlights how these two factors are directly targeted, building on the rationale for the cognitive model in general. A brief handout for the rationale that you can share with patients is presented in Handout 1.

Therapist: Okay, so we have spoken in general about reducing emotional intensity through cognitive, behavioral, and physical strategies, but let's talk more specifically about how this relates to PTSD. I think it can be helpful to start with an example from the past week of a time when you noticed feeling particularly triggered by a reminder of the bus accident [the index trauma that brought the patient into treatment]. Can you think of an example like that?

Patient: I mean it happens constantly. I was late to work this week, and my partner was telling me that I should just take the bus instead of walking—I've been walking 45 minutes instead of taking the bus because I'm just terrified to get on one again. When my partner suggested that I just take the bus, I flipped out.

Therapist: This is the perfect example. Try to put yourself back in that moment when you were upset for a moment to jog your memory.

What thoughts were going through your mind that made it make perfect sense for you to "flip out" at your partner's suggestion?

Patient: I just remember feeling so upset and angry.

Therapist: Right, those are the emotions that you were feeling: anger and maybe some other things too. What must you have been telling yourself to make those emotions make sense?

Patient: I guess I was thinking that my partner just does not get it—I'm terrified that if I get on a bus again, we'll get in another accident, and I won't be so lucky next time.

Therapist: Now I'm starting to understand—so you had at least two important thoughts in that moment. One was about the probability that something horrible will happen again, which your PTSD tells you is likely, given what you went through. The second is feeling like other people, specifically your partner, just don't get it. These are both examples of trauma-related cognitions, in this case about the world in general and about other people not understanding you.

Patient: Yes, plus also: you never know what's going on for a driver on a given day! And it's not just the bus drivers; they are probably the safer ones on the road. It's everyone else. Something unpredictable could happen at any time, and before you know it - it's too late.

Therapist: Thank you for sharing those examples - it's helpful to hear about how these trauma-related cognitions had a major impact on you during what was already a stressful moment of being late for work. What did you choose to do in that situation?

Patient: Well, for a moment I was thinking that maybe I should just "suck it up" and take the bus because I was worried I would be fired if I'm late again. But then I thought better of it and decided to just pay five times as much as the bus fare on a taxi. That was probably a stupid decision financially, but it made sense emotionally.

Therapist: What you experienced is so common among patients who are suffering from PTSD. The anxiety and distress that the symptoms cause encourage people to avoid reminders of their trauma. In the short term, that avoidance tends to decrease anxiety and allow for the person to feel some relief. In the long term, though, avoidance tends to destroy self-confidence and increase anxiety. What has your experience been of avoidance?

Patient: I sort of hate to admit it, but I mean I'm more afraid now of just living then I've ever been. It feels like since the accident happened, I'm doing less and less things every week but feeling more and more afraid. So, I suppose that's sort of proof of what you are talking about.

Therapist: Yes, what you described is exactly what we see in folks who are suffering with PTSD, and it can feel so disheartening. The good news is that the treatment that we are going to do together is designed exactly to help interrupt this pattern. Is it okay with you if I tell you a bit about how?

Patient: Yes, I'd like to learn more about it.

Therapist: In our treatment, we're going to start with a behavioral intervention to reduce this pattern as quickly as possible. We have four types of behavioral strategies that we can use, three of which are focused on reducing anxiety and one of which is focused on reducing depression.

The three anxiety-focused strategies all include different types of exposure strategies. Have you ever heard of exposure therapy?

Patient: Sort of – like if someone is afraid of spiders, they have to hold a tarantula or something?

Therapist: That's exactly right. Exposure therapy is based on the idea that if you do the thing that anxiety tells you to do (avoid), anxiety will worsen over time. Conversely, if you do the opposite of what anxiety tells you to do (approach), anxiety will decrease. We have three different types of exposures that I'll tell you all about when the time comes. In a nutshell, these exposures might be to people, places, situations, memories, or physical sensations that are objectively safe, but that you have been avoiding since the trauma. Importantly, you'll always be in charge of this process, and I'm never going to pressure you to do things that you don't feel ready to do. People who do exposures tend to find that they feel much more in control of their emotions, and much more confident in general about their sense of power over their lives. Do you have any questions about that so far?

Patient: I have a million questions, but mostly I just want to say that it sounds really scary.

Therapist: I hear you – I promise that we will set things up for you to set the pace that feels right for you. But also, if you were thrilled about the idea of doing exposures, we probably wouldn't need to do them at all. I have a handout [Give the patient Handout 2] that goes through some common questions and answers for folks who are beginning exposure therapy that I'll give to you.

Patient: You're probably right – I probably wouldn't need to be in therapy if this were easy to do.

Therapist: Exactly. The last behavioral strategy that we might do is about trying to build more opportunities for doing things that make you feel good about yourself. We call it "behavioral activation," and research shows that it can really help with depression, which is super common among people with PTSD. If it's relevant to you, we'll talk more about it later. Do you have any questions so far?

Patient: How much work is this going to be?

Therapist: Good question: It will be quite a bit of work, both in session together and between sessions. We'll have you do exercises between sessions to get the most out of the treatment. Since we typically only meet for a shorter duration of around 12 sessions or so, we want to make the most of our time together. How does that sound to you?

Patient: I get it. It took me a while to get to this place, so it's going to take effort to get me out of it.

Therapist: There's one more thing that I want to tell you about, which is focusing on trauma-related cognitions. With everything that we do together, we're going to be paying attention to the way that you are seeing yourself, other people, and the world in general to highlight how these cognitions are an ever-present part of your suffering from PTSD. The more that we can build awareness of them, the more options you have for responding to them differently.
So that's the overall description of the treatment. As we get to each of the areas that we'll be working on, I'll give you a thorough explanation about why and how we do them. Do you have any questions now?

Note that this rationale covers several core components of CBT for PTSD. It covers principles of exposure, the fact that there are multiple kinds of exposure, a brief rationale for why exposure can be helpful, a brief description of behavioral activation, and an overview of a focus on trauma-related cognitions throughout. This foundation can help a patient to give informed consent about the treatment plan, but also to make sure that they are not overwhelmed with information before they begin.

Important Considerations for the Rationale for CBT

When a patient presents for therapy for the first time, they are typically feeling nervous and on edge. As a result, it can be easy for them to get distracted during the rationale and only half hear what the therapist is explaining. This is normal, even when therapists explain the treatment very clearly. For this reason, in prolonged exposure (PE; Foa et al., 2007, 2019) therapy, clinicians provide information to patients in multiple formats, including verbally, in written form, and in audio-recording form by recording the session for the patient to review later. By presenting the important information in multiple formats, a patient has a better chance of consolidating the information after the session if consolidation does not occur in session.

Sometimes therapists who are newer to this model of therapy are reluctant to engage in a conversation that feels didactic in nature, especially if the therapist usually practices supportive or psychodynamic therapy. To cope with this discomfort, the therapist might skirt the psychoeducation section, which means that they miss the opportunity to share essential information with their patient. This is particularly likely when a newer therapist perceives that aspects of the psychoeducation are "obvious," and therefore unnecessary to discuss with the patient. While the therapist might be an expert on PTSD and mental health, the patient might have very little experience of therapy or psychiatric illnesses and may greatly benefit from a thorough explanation from a trustworthy messenger. Even more problematic is a scenario in which a patient has been given misinformation from an unreliable source and the therapist misses an opportunity to correct that misinformation. Thus, it is essential to ensure that the therapist takes their time with psychoeducation and does not attempt to rush the process.

Another common roadblock related to the rationale for CBT for PTSD is the tendency for a therapist who is newer to this model to lean too heavily on rationale to the exclusion of rapport building or another important intervention. As is discussed in Chapter 6 in the context of processing exposures, therapists occasionally default into didactic mode when they are anxious. For instance, if the therapist does not know what to say, they might default to psychoeducation. Or if a patient is very emotionally upset, the therapist might inadvertently shift into psychoeducation mode to deescalate the intensity of the emotions in the room. While psychoeducation is extremely important, the goal of psychoeducation should never be to reduce emotional expression. Nevertheless, newer therapists occasionally notice that as emotional intensity increases in the room, or if they are feeling unsure of themselves for whatever reason, they might default to psychoeducation when other strategies (e.g., validation, active listening, continuing the activity that was already underway) are more appropriate. When getting to know the patient, it is essential to pepper in psychoeducation in a conversational manner so that the therapist makes sure to take sufficient time with it but also keeps the psychoeducation provision conversational. The best psychoeducation conversation builds on the real-world experiences of the patient and uses those experiences to highlight how PTSD is maintained and how it can be treated.

Getting Buy-in Around the Idea of Exposures

Some therapists appreciate the structure and skills-based focus of CBT for PTSD but are reluctant to implement exposures as an element of their treatment, especially imaginal exposures. I discuss this topic in detail in Chapter 6. When therapists have a bias *against* exposure for PTSD, this can steer patients away from exposure and toward other CBT strategies that are perceived as less emotionally evocative, especially cognitive strategies. Therapists should explore their biases about any aspect of the treatment approach before they begin their psychoeducation and rationale discussion with patients and attempt to reduce the impact of their bias on how they communicate about treatment options.

Some therapists feel strongly that patients should be presented with a menu of options for their treatment and be empowered to select the ingredients for their treatment plan. This can generally be a successful strategy, with the caveat that a clinician who is biased against exposures may be more likely to inadvertently guide their patients away from them. For instance, therapists might describe exposure practice as "extremely difficult" or use other language that casts the effective therapeutic technique in a negative light. These therapists may find that their patients are opting out of exposure-based approaches to CBT and then use that selection as further confirmation that exposure therapy is not palatable to patients. Patients should have control over their treatment, and that control should be provided with unbiased recommendations about the full package of treatment options to allow for genuine informed consent.

In Chapters 5 and 6, I provide a detailed rationale for *in vivo* and imaginal exposures, respectively. Those rationales are to be used in the sessions in which the exposure practice is being introduced. In earlier sessions of the treatment plan, the language that the therapist selects to introduce exposure practice is extremely important. We must balance providing accurate information to allow our patients to know what to expect, while not exacerbating anticipatory anxiety about a practice that will begin several weeks later. The language that I use in early psychoeducation sessions for *in vivo* exposure usually focuses on helping patients to grow their lives in whatever direction is important to them. I inform patients that the goal of *in vivo* exposure is to understand how the trauma has changed their sense of control over what they can and cannot do, and to allow them to regain that control by nudging themselves to do things that are objectively safe and yet feel "off-limits" since the trauma. In early treatment sessions, I inform patients that imaginal exposure allows them to tell the story of what happened to them in a safe and nonjudgmental atmosphere, while allowing them to feel whatever they need to feel about their experiences. When framed with this language, most patients tend to agree that these exposure practices are necessary for their healing process, even if they are nervous about embarking on them. I remind patients that the trepidation that they feel about exposure practice is a very helpful indicator that it is exactly what we should be doing to help them in their therapeutic journey. I often say to patients, *If you were not nervous to do exposure practice, we probably would not need to do it in the first place. The fact that you are a bit nervous about it tells us that we are heading in the right direction.*

Summary

Providing the rationale for CBT for PTSD allows patients and therapists alike to make sure that they are on the same page before formally commencing the therapy. It can help to provide psychoeducation about the cognitive model (i.e., the association among thoughts, behaviors, and physical sensations in the context of difficult emotions). The cognitive model makes obvious that there are options for interventions that directly address cognitions, behaviors, or physical sensations, and that depending on the patient's symptom profile, you might consider each of those types of interventions. Then, it can help to inform patients that CBT for PTSD tends to emphasize a reduction in avoidance and trauma-related cognitions, given that these symptom types are fundamental to the development and maintenance of PTSD. You can also share with patients that there is an option to use strategies to target depression and responding to uncomfortable physical sensations as needed. As therapists provide psychoeducation and the therapeutic rationale to patients, it is essential to have awareness of any biases about treatment components, as patients are likely to pick up on those biases and make their treatment plan decisions on that basis. Therapists should balance providing necessary information for patients to know what to expect in CBT for PTSD with ensuring that patients feel empowered to do the treatment, even if their confidence is rattled.

5 Optimizing *in Vivo* Exposure

As mentioned in Chapters 1 and 2, avoidance is a core and central feature of PTSD (Schuettler & Boals, 2011; Sheynin et al., 2017). Longitudinal research suggests that avoidance predicts the onset and maintenance of PTSD symptoms (Marx & Sloan, 2005). Given the centrality of avoidance in PTSD, in exposure therapy, patients practice *approaching* reminders of the trauma. *In vivo* (real-world) exposure practices are appropriate when an individual with PTSD reports that they are avoiding concrete stimuli that remind the person of the trauma or feel more dangerous since the trauma occurred.

How to Introduce *in Vivo* Exposure to Patients With PTSD

At the point wherein you are introducing *in vivo* exposure practices to your patient, they have likely already been introduced to the overall rationale for CBT (see Chapter 4). Most commonly, patients are terrified about the prospect of completing an exposure practice even if they intellectually understand its value. It is essential to revisit the rationale to justify *in vivo* exposure before getting started. Glossing over the rationale is common in therapists who are new to this approach, and they will commonly report, "We already talked about this at the beginning of therapy." Patients with PTSD often experience high-intensity emotions in early therapy sessions, which may make it challenging to encode, consolidate, and recall new information (Dickie et al., 2008; van Marle, 2015). This is one of the reasons why patients with PTSD commonly report challenges with tasks involving concentration and working memory (Litz & Keane, 1989) – existing in a baseline state of high-intensity emotions makes it hard to focus. For this reason, it is essential to remind the patient about the goals of *in vivo* exposure practice before getting started. By prioritizing the rationale, the patient can provide informed consent for the practice and stay in control of the pacing of their *in vivo* practices. Always position yourselves so that the patient is in the metaphorical driver's seat and you are holding the map.

Here is an example script for how to introduce or reintroduce the rationale for *in vivo* exposure practice for PTSD using hypothetical examples from the patient's prior assessment.

Therapist: We're at the point in therapy where I think it would be really useful to turn our attention toward growing your life in the directions that you think matter to you. You shared with me that there are several situations that you avoid since the trauma happened because they remind you of what happened or because they now feel more dangerous. For instance, you told me that you stopped going to school events with your son since the rape because they are crowded and there are unfamiliar men around. When you told me about this, I could tell it was painful to discuss. Why does this topic bring on intense emotions for you?

Patient: I'm so torn because, on the one hand, I want to be there for my son – he's my whole world, and I want to support him. On the other hand, I start to panic when I'm in groups with a lot of people, especially if there are men there whom I don't know. It takes me back to that night of the rape. I start hyperventilating and feel like I'm going to lose it. No one wants to see that. So, I just decided I would stop going. But now I feel like such a loser of a parent.

Therapist: Thank you for sharing that – I can see the pain in your eyes when you talk about it here again. I'm hearing that it's terrifying to be at these school events, and that it's also important to go so that you can be there for your son, and because it's taking a toll on your self-esteem. I could see how it feels like you're backed up against a wall.

At this part in therapy, our goal is to help you get unstuck. These *in vivo* (or real-world) exposures often help people to get unstuck. Would you be willing for me to tell you about how *in vivo* exposure works?

Patient: You can tell me, but no promises that I'll do it.

Therapist: I hear you. Like you, I wouldn't commit to something unless I knew what I was getting into. The goal for *in vivo* exposure is to get some data about situations that you are tempted to avoid because of the PTSD. You could think of this like setting up experiments. Through trial and error, people tend to find that they are more capable of doing things than they thought and more capable of tolerating their emotional reactions in those situations. Some people find that their intense emotions decrease over time, too.

If you agree to move forward with this, we'll follow a straightforward plan. First, we will make a list of situations that stir up high-intensity emotions, and we'll use a handout to help us [Handout 3]. Second, we will discuss your hypotheses, or predictions, about what you think might happen in those situations. Some of those hypotheses might be about how anxious or upset you might feel in the situation, and some might be about what you are telling yourself will happen in that situation. Third, you and I will collaboratively plan the experiment you are willing to do for the first exposure. Fourth, we do the experiments – sometimes we might do some together, and sometimes you'll do them on your own. Fifth, we discuss what you learned – what did your data show, and did your hypothesis come true? Do you have any questions about this so far?

Patient: This seems pretty straightforward in theory, but I'm really nervous about it already.

Therapist: I'm glad that it makes intuitive sense to you, and it's very common for people to feel nervous about it before we start. There are two ground rules I want to make clear before we decide if you'd like to proceed. First, I'm never going to ask you to do anything that is objectively unsafe. Second, I'm never going to trick or coerce you into doing something that you're not willing to do. In my experience, these *in vivo* exposures only work if the person doing them (you) is in control. Any questions?

Patient: I'm just confused because it's not like I'm never in scary situations – I find myself in them all the time. That's why I stopped leaving my house so much. I was getting triggered everywhere I went! How was that not an *in vivo* exposure?

Therapist: That's such a good point. What we know is that going into scary situations does not promote new learning if the person escapes from the situation as soon as possible. For instance, if you went to a school event, started hyperventilating, and then said, "I'm about to do something out of control, I'm getting out of here!" then there was not an opportunity to learn about your ability to tolerate high anxiety without it affecting your behavior (in this case, without it making you "lose control," whatever that means, and we'll talk about that). For this reason, we must be careful in setting up the experiments so that you can get the most out of them. What do you think about that?

Patient: I could see how that makes sense, but it's still really awful. I wish I didn't have to do this.

Therapist: I can tell that this is really frightening. My guess is that if you didn't feel this way – if this were actually really easy – we probably wouldn't need to do it. I'm sensing that because this is really intimidating, it might be really important to try it. At the end of the day, it's completely up to you to decide. What do you think?

Patient: Yeah, I mean coming to therapy in the first place has been awful (no offense!) because I just hate talking about how my life is in shambles. I have to do something to get my life back, so I feel like I'll try anything at this point.

Therapist: I'm really proud of you – it's not easy to decide that, but you did anyway. I think this could really help. Let's dive in, then.

Planning for *in Vivo* Exposures

Expert exposure therapists vary in their recommendations about the optimal order of operations for *in vivo* exposure preparations. In prolonged exposure (PE) therapy (Foa et al., 2007, 2019), the recommended approach is to begin by introducing patients to a scale for assessing anticipated or actual distress for an exposure, the Subjective Units of Distress Scale (SUDS). Then anchor points are identified based on past experiences in which the patient engaged in an activity that made them feel a range of SUDs values (typically 0, 50, and 100 at a minimum). The objective of these anchor points is to assist the patient in having prior experiences by which to compare their expected SUDs for a given *in vivo* exposure. Next, participants brainstorm a list of 10–15 items to add to an exposure hierarchy *without* rating them. After that, each item is given an expected SUDs rating. In other CBT for PTSD approaches, hierarchy building has fewer steps. For instance, in the Unified Protocol (Gallagher, 2017), participants simply brainstorm the list of avoided items, rate how much distress and avoidance are associated with each item, and begin exposure to them, with explicit encouragement not to do the items in a predetermined order (Barlow, Farchione, et al., 2017). These two approaches to generating an *in vivo* exposure hierarchy have not been directly compared. Given that multiple approaches recommend orienting patients to SUDs and brainstorming/rating the list, only those two components are described here.

Introduction to Subjective Units of Distress (SUDs)

In CBT for PTSD, SUDs are the method for communication about levels of distress. SUDs ratings are made to plan the order of exposures and to reflect upon how distressing the exposure was after it is completed. Of note, distress is intentionally broad; for some patients, SUDs are synonymous with anxiety, whereas for other patients, SUDs can include a combination of multiple emotions (e.g., shame, anger, anxiety, guilt). Usually, a 0–100 point scale is indicated, where 100 is the most distress that a person could possibly feel and 0 is a complete absence of distress. For some patients, a 100-point scale is too overwhelming, which detracts from the exposure. In those cases, patients can consider a simpler scale (0–10) or, as is discussed in *Prolonged Exposure Therapy for Adolescents* (Foa et al., 2009) and in *Coping Cat* (Rifkin et al., 2021), a visual depiction can be useful (e.g., a feelings thermometer). The scale itself is trivial – SUDs are intended to serve as a tool to promote communication between the patient and therapist about their distress as they anticipate an exposure or complete one. A common mistake for early therapists is to become hyperfocused on SUDs values as the sole barometer of success in treatment, which results in missed information about other key indicators (functioning, quality of life, social connection, etc.) that are essential for gauging treatment outcome.

Brainstorming an *in Vivo* Exposure Practice List

It is always easiest to start building the experiment list (hierarchy) based on the content that emerged when you were conducting your diagnostic evaluation with the patient. Given that avoidance is assessed during the evaluation, you will likely already have some ideas about things that the patient is avoiding. Building the hierarchy almost always takes longer than anticipated. I typically approach hierarchy building as a first draft, knowing that we will revisit the hierarchy repeatedly throughout treatment. It is not necessary to conclude the hierarchy building session feeling like you have a beautiful treatment plan. Instead, the first hierarchy is a starting point in treatment planning. For that reason, prioritize being responsive to your patient in the hierarchybuilding process rather than prioritizing building the perfect hierarchy.

I usually first list an item or two that the patient has already discussed as something that they avoid. Then, I turn it over to the patient with an open-ended prompt and give them some time to sit with it (e.g., *What else should go on here?*). Prioritize items that the patient generates and praise them for disclosing them. This is a vulnerable (sometimes even emotionally painful) task, and it would be so much easier to lie! It is extremely brave to be forthcoming, and we can build our patients' trust by being excited about their active participation and openly acknowledging it. For example, I'll praise my patients by saying, *I'm so glad you told me about that one, I really appreciate your honesty. I know it can feel vulnerable to open up about these situations – good for you for doing it anyway.*

As a general note, many new therapists struggle with providing enough praise in therapy or with delivering sufficient warmth and genuineness in their praise. The best way to get data on this is to watch tapes of yourself during these interactions. I have often thought, *I'm being so supportive!* in my sessions and then, when I watch it back, I realize that the interaction was a 3/10 on the support scale (where 10 is oozing warmth and support and 0 is cold and detached). It is tricky to calibrate the right intensity of praise until you get more experience – watch and learn from your successes, and above all, slow down and stick with your patients. This allows you to capture moments to praise and to really be *with them* (not a step ahead) as they do this work.

Rating the *in Vivo* Exposure Practice List

Whether or not ratings are collected after the entire hierarchy is generated (as is recommended in PE therapy) or after each item is generated is up for debate. Some expert exposure therapists report that it is more efficient to wait until the list is generated in its entirety before rating items on it because then patients are better able to gauge the difficulty of each item relative to the others. Other expert exposure therapists report that it feels more seamless to rate the items as the hierarchy is being generated, as doing so can inform whether there is a need to focus on items that are much more or less difficult. The ideal hierarchy includes the following:

- Items across a wide range of SUDs
- Items that can be repeated
- Items that are in the control of the patient
- Items that do not require other people

Not all hierarchy items will meet these criteria, but many items should. As is recommended in PE therapy (Foa et al., 2007, 2019), if the list is filled with items that are all too high or too low, the therapist can prompt, "What would make this item more difficult? What would make it less difficult?"

Subtle variations in contextual factors affect learning during exposure practice (Bouton, 1988). For example, environmental factors, such as time of day, may have a major impact on expected SUDs for a given patient. Varying the presence of social supports can also have a major impact on SUDs. In some cases, varying internal factors (e.g., fatigue, coffee consumption, clothing choices for altering temperature control) also alter SUDs levels. Each of these contextual factors should be considered when planning exposures.

"Finishing" the *in Vivo* Exposure Hierarchy

As mentioned previously, it is rare to conclude a hierarchy building session with a *perfect* hierarchy. Even very experienced therapists find that generating a solid hierarchy is extremely time-consuming – it almost always takes longer than anticipated. New therapists often put unnecessary pressure on themselves (and on patients) to approach the hierarchy as a firm plan to guide the remaining therapy sessions. Instead, the hierarchy should be treated as a work in progress to be revisited frequently throughout therapy for new additions and deletions as indicated. When the *in vivo* hierarchy is introduced, a realistic objective is to walk away from the conversation with one or two items that the patient could begin practicing.

In PE therapy (Foa et al., 2007, 2019) and in the Unified Protocol (Barlow, Sauer-Zavala, et al., 2017), patients are explicitly assigned to review the hierarchy as part of their homework. At a minimum, in the session after the hierarchy is introduced, it is good practice to revisit the hierarchy and inquire about whether the patient has any new ideas or changes to make since the last session. From there on, patients will commonly volunteer new exposure ideas based on what has been working and where they feel increased confidence (or realized new sources of avoidance).

Agreeing on the First *in Vivo* Practice

Remembering that our role in CBT is that of a coach, the process for selecting the first *in vivo* exposure practice should occur in a collaborative fashion. Activities that are generated by the patient are much more likely to be tied to the patient's overarching goals and values and should ideally take priority. The selection of the first *in vivo* exposure practice must balance multiple considerations, namely: factors that will impact adherence; repetition potential; emotional intensity and learning; drop-out risk; subsequent exposure planning; patient's perceptions of therapist beliefs about their capabilities; and patient's perceptions of their own capabilities, as described in Table 2.

Given this balancing act, it is helpful to plan a first exposure in the medium to medium-low range (30–50 on a 100-point SUDS). We will often recommend selecting two exposure items that could each be repeated at least three times before the next therapy session. For both exposure practices, it is essential to identify the patient's expectation for the exposure in advance (in other words, what the patient is most worried will happen during the exposure). It is also essential to concretize the exposure in terms of the setting, duration, time of day, and other critical factors in advance.

As is typical in other CBT approaches, it is ideal to check in with the patient about the likelihood that they will complete an exposure before ending the session. As described elsewhere (Cully & Teten, 2008), one way to gauge the likelihood of success is to ask patients to rate their confidence (0–100%, where 100% is "I'm certain I will do it" and 0% is "It's not going to happen") that they will complete both exposure practices at least three times before the next therapy session. If the patient's confidence rating is less than 80%,

Table 2. The impact of in vivo exposure practices that are too difficult or too easy

Theme	Items that are too difficult	Items that are too easy
Adherence	The patient will not do the exercise because it is too difficult ("I can't handle doing that").	The patient will not do the exercise because it is too easy ("What is the point of doing this?").
Repetition potential	Even if the patient does the activity once, it is less likely that they will repeat the activity because it was *too difficult*.	Even if the patient does the activity once, it is less likely that they will repeat the activity because it was *too easy*.
Emotional intensity and learning	Even if the patient completes the activity, they might become overwhelmed with negative emotions, which could prevent them from future practice.	The patient does not become emotionally engaged in the exercise, which prevents learning.
Dropout risk	A patient who becomes too overwhelmed by the exercise might drop out of treatment.	The patient feels like the therapist missed the mark or is not going to be helpful, and therefor drops out of treatment.
Subsequent exposures	The patient compensates by reducing willingness to move on to the next item on the hierarchy.	The patient compensates and starts pushing themselves to do exercises that are far too difficult during the next exposure.
Therapist perceptions (according to the patient)	The patient feels ashamed that they cannot do what the therapist asks and therefore feels less connected to the therapist.	The patient feels patronized, or like the therapist is not aware of their strengths, and feels less connected to the therapist.
Patient perceptions	Self-esteem is reduced due to an unsuccessful exposure (especially if the patient escapes or decides not to repeat the exercise).	The patient has missed an opportunity to build self-esteem or empowerment by practicing challenging exercises.

you might consider downshifting the exposure intensity by inquiring, *What would make this easier?* and changing the activity or by identifying barriers to success and problem solving around them. Some experts suggest an even lower bar to prompt a change in assignment (i.e., a 60% or lower rating). It might also be important to attend to elevated confidence ratings (i.e., 100% confidence), which could indicate that the task is too easy or that the patient is not realistically considering potential obstacles, to allow for adjustment of the task accordingly.

Reinforcing Exposure Practice

Completed Homework

The (rare) patient who presents with a fully completed homework list should be applauded. Patients who have been avoiding reminders of their trauma must draw on enormous courage and motivation to complete their exposure therapy homework, and these accomplishments should be made very explicit and celebrated!

Partial Homework Completion

Despite their best intentions to complete their *in vivo* homework (or any exposure homework, for that matter), patients often present with partial homework completion. For many of our patients, homework practice conjures up memories of shameful experiences in school, with finger-wagging teachers expressing disappointment at their forgetfulness, lack of commitment, or mistakes. The association between homework and ridicule is often strong and can cause patients to experience strong shame reactions when discussing imperfect homework completion. For some, discomfort with nonperfect performance can be so intense that they cancel their future therapy appointments to prevent discussing their perceived "failure." My motto for homework adherence is: Ask for what you want to see, take whatever you can get, and praise the heck out of it. It is hard to provide excessive praise, especially for patients with PTSD, who often struggle with disempowerment and low self-esteem (Adams & Boscarino, 2006).

Reinforcing homework completion shares principles with other types of reinforcement. Labeled praise is optimal. For instance, rather than a vague *I'm glad you did some homework*, it is preferable to offer specific feedback on what is impressive about their homework, coupled with an opportunity to play Monday-morning quarterback in reflecting on the success. For example:

> *I'm really impressed that you were able to get yourself to do* [homework task] – *I would imagine it was hard to build up the courage to do it that day, and it would have been easier to not do it at all. How did you get yourself to do that?*

Patients with PTSD are often extremely hard on themselves and quickly minimize the significance of their achievements. It can be helpful to highlight this process when it occurs. For example:

> *I notice that as I'm telling you, "I'm proud of you for doing the* in vivo *exposure," your response is downplaying it and making it seem like no big deal. From where I'm sitting, it's a* huge *deal that you got yourself to do something*

you've been avoiding for [months? years? decades?]. *What's going through your mind about this?*

Here, I am attempting to elicit the cognition that directly predicts "minimizing accomplishment" behavior. It might also be important to elicit the emotional contributor to that behavior as well (e.g., "What are you feeling when you say that it's no big deal?") Either way, this allows us to build a mini-cognitive model on how even an accomplishment can be punishing, as described in Figure 1.

Building this cognitive model (and drawing it out whenever possible) can help to highlight how punishing good behavior makes it less likely for the behavior to occur. When a patient accomplishes their homework practice (even partially) but follows this with negative self-talk about how they should have done it *years ago*, or how they should have done *more*, it reduces the likelihood that they will do future homework. Thus, it is essential to increase patients' awareness of this pattern when it emerges. Then, it is essential to have the patient practice acknowledging and celebrating their accomplishments with homework completion going forward. Patients with PTSD often need guidance and coaching on this, and if you offer labeled, genuine praise, a critical learning opportunity emerges.

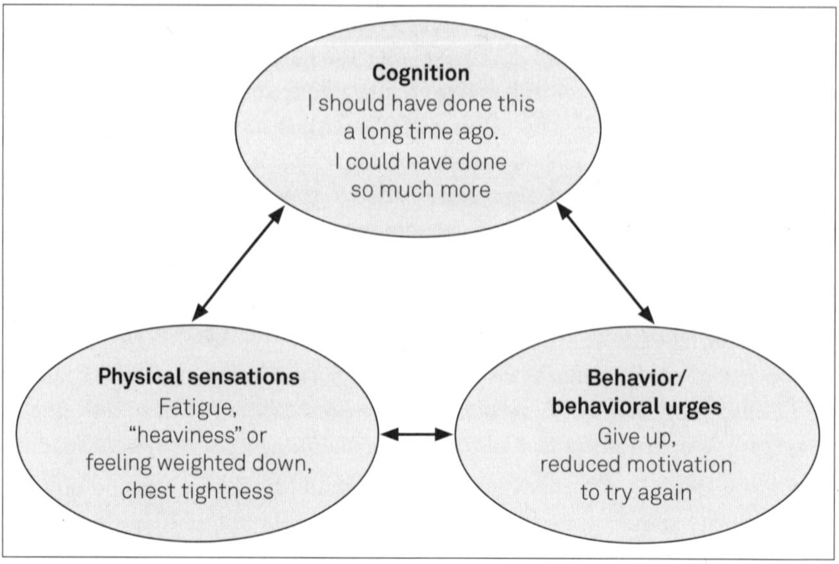

Figure 1. Cognitive model describing a patient who minimizes an accomplishment

No Homework Completion

As with every treatment modality that includes homework, patients with PTSD will occasionally not complete any of their homework goals. As with nonperfect homework completion, a lack of any homework completion sometimes results in patients skipping the session, or even dropping out of treatment altogether. If the patient cancels for a nonobvious reason (illness, an accident, a family matter), I like to arrange to speak to the patient briefly at the time that we were originally scheduled to meet. If the patient emails to cancel, I usually respond with an expression of care and concern and recommend a 5-minute check-in call at the start of our scheduled time if possible. This check-in call allows for a brief assessment of the reason why the patient canceled the session.

When you learn that a lack of homework completion was the primary driver of canceling, I start with validation and normalizing, such as by saying, I'm really glad you shared that with me. It is often really difficult for folks to do *in vivo* exposure practices – if this was easy, you probably wouldn't need to be in this therapy.

Then I try to schedule a new appointment as soon as possible, with an invitation to come to that appointment even if they have not done any of the homework. Sometimes giving permission to skip the homework between now and the new session time will increase the likelihood that the patient will come to the next session. This is a good short-term strategy to promote engagement, but with obvious downsides of minimizing the perceived importance of homework; however, a patient who never comes back to therapy is also never going to do more therapy homework. The priority in these dilemmas is usually keeping the patient engaged at the expense of losing some credibility about homework. If the patient seems motivated to "get back on the horse" of homework practice, I like to play devil's advocate, such as by saying *I'm so excited that you want to get back in the swing of homework, but maybe what we set out to do was too much this time. Should we make the goal a bit less intense?*

If the patient comes to their therapy session, they might present with complicated emotions. Some patients are riddled with shame ("I'm never going to be able to do anything right. Ever since the trauma, I have been incapable of making good decisions"); others are angry with themselves or with the therapist ("I came here to feel better and you set me up to feel worse!"); and still others feel overcome with anxiety ("I'm too scared to do what you're asking me to do") or sadness and hopelessness ("Nothing is ever going to get better for me – what's the point in trying?"). When strong emotions enter the room, it is always helpful to start by celebrating that the patient came to the session at all, for instance: *I can tell you are feeling really strong [emotion] today, and I'm guessing you might have been tempted to not come at all. I'm really glad you're here so that we can figure this out together. Thanks for coming back.*

After acknowledging and validating the emotion, there are multiple paths forward (see Table 3). The "deal with it later" path is appropriate when you have other essential treatment components to enact in the session. One example would be if the treatment plan necessitates prioritizing imaginal exposure and you might be willing to discuss *in vivo* exposure adherence after the imaginal exposure is completed for the session. The downside of this path is

Table 3. Paths to take when a patient with PTSD has not completed any of their *in vivo* homework

Path type	When you might use this	Downsides	Priority
Deal with it later	You have other priorities for the session that will be sacrificed if a lot of time is dedicated to homework adherence.	By spending less time discussing ways to improve homework adherence, it is less likely to improve on its own. It also reduces the credibility of the homework because it communicates that it is "no big deal" if the homework is not completed.	Keeping the patient moving forward.
Make it a big deal	When the patient has repeatedly come to sessions without doing any homework; at this point, the "elephant in the room" is that it is silly to continue assigning homework if it will not be completed.	This discussion sometimes leads to a mutual decision to end therapy early.	Preserving fidelity to the treatment and treatment credibility.
Acknowledge it	When you want to draw attention to the lack of homework completion and express concern about it to the patient.	When a patient is emotionally dysregulated or had a crisis, it can feel invalidating or shaming even to acknowledge the lack of homework completion.	Keeping the patient moving forward and increasing the credibility of homework in the PTSD treatment.

that credibility about homework is reduced because if you assign a task that is not completed and do not follow up, the patient may assume that it was not important in the first place. Another path, the "make it a big deal path", can be appropriate when there are repeated instances of patients presenting for sessions without having completed their homework. One of my favorite supervisors, Dr. Lynn McFarr, always framed this approach as "What kind of a therapist would I be if I didn't talk about the fact that homework is not happening here?" The priority of this path is in preserving fidelity to the treatment protocol; a patient is *not* receiving an adequate dose of therapy if the requisite homework is not happening. If we continue the therapy when homework is not happening, we risk damaging the credibility of the therapy altogether and enhancing the risk that a patient has a nonhelpful experience with therapy and then believes that "no therapy will ever work for me." In some cases, taking the perspective that homework nonadherence is a big deal necessitates opening the door to ending therapy prematurely. There are circumstances where a mutual decision to end therapy early is an optimal outcome, including when a patient is regularly not engaging in the tasks recommended by the therapy.

Highlighting the Learning From the Exposure

The aim of every exposure practice is to create new learning or reinforce adaptive learning. One way to highlight new learning is to evaluate whether *expectation violation* occurred. In other words, did the patient's explicit expectation (recorded before the exposure practice) occur? What were the data to support or refute the expectation? It is essential to assist the patient in recognizing the difference between what they expected to occur versus what occurred during the exposure practice. Those differences may be indicated in terms of feared aversive outcomes (e.g., the person will yell at me; I will be rejected), a change in distress as indicated by SUDs, or the ability to perform a certain task after completing the exposure (when the patient perceives that their anxiety will interfere with functioning).

In some cases, exposures will not go according to plan. Even exposures with aversive outcomes can create opportunities for learning about the patient's ability to survive another awful situation (which can be important when patients with PTSD feel disempowered). When the therapist approaches exposure practices as experiments for new learning, the patient can try new strategies for dealing with anxiety. Even if one strategy does not feel like an optimal fit for the patient, this provides both the patient and the therapist with new data about how to move forward. For these reasons, even nonideal exposures are still helpful to the therapy process.

Helping Patients to Stay in the Present Moment

When you observe a patient as they complete an *in vivo* exposure practice, there are several core objectives that include: helping the patient to stay in the present moment; optimizing learning; following through on the completion of the exposure; supporting the patient in reducing safety behaviors and modulating emotional intensity; celebrating wins; and supporting the patient in consolidation of learning. As detailed in Table 4, there are predictable challenges that emerge with each of these goals, and the table describes tips for anticipating and overcoming those challenges to promote successful exposure practice.

Reducing the Focus on SUDs

Emotional processing theory (Foa & Kozak, 1986) proposed that within-session habituation (or reduction in anxiety within an exposure session) was essential for learning, a finding that has some support in the literature (de Kleine et al., 2017). However, some studies have refuted this claim (Bluett et al., 2014) and highlight that SUDs are not especially meaningful indicators of treatment progress. New therapists often become overly fixated on SUDs to guide their next exposure practice. Too much focus on SUDS misses the point of exposure practice – new learning. New learning can occur even without a significant change in SUDs within or between exposure practices. For this reason, therapists should consider a few key tips to guide the success of the exposure, regardless of SUDs:

- *Get concrete:* Concretize the parameters of the exposure before it occurs. Specify the location, time of day, duration, and presence/absence of other people or safety objects. Also, specify how many times the patient should practice the exposure between the current session and the next session.
- *Use expectation violation as a guiding principle:* Every exposure practice should occur only after the therapist and patient are clear on the patient's hypothesis for the exposure. In other words, what does the patient expect will occur? In the worst-case scenario, what does the patient fear will happen? Typically, expectations for exposures are about an aversive event occurring, high anxiety that will never subside, or an inability to tolerate anxiety (leading to lack of behavioral control). These hypotheses should be elicited and written down before the exposure. After the exposure, the therapist should explore whether the hypothesis was supported and with what data. Expectation violation, a core mechanism of action of exposure therapy, occurs when there is a difference between what the patient expected to occur and what occurred.

Table 4. Objectives when observing an *in vivo* exposure practice

Topic	Goal	Challenges	Tips
Present moment awareness	Assist the patient to stay in the present moment.	The patient engages in distraction, talks about unrelated topics, or jumps into discussions about what's to come later.	Observe and describe what you are noticing (e.g., *It seems like we have gotten out of the exposure – let's jump back in. Talk me through what we're doing here.*).
Optimizing learning during the exposure	Support the patient in gathering the data necessary to support/violate their expectancies.	The patient engages in post-hoc hypotheses ("I knew this wouldn't be hard all along").	Direct the patient to gather data (and track that data) about the actual outcome(s) of the exposure.
Following through on the exposure	Coach the patient to initiate and complete the agreed upon exposure.	The patient struggles to get started, refuses to start, or wants to end the exposure prematurely.	Make warm and supportive but directive coaching statements about starting the exposure (*I know that you can do this. Let's go ahead and begin*), sticking with the exposure (*I can tell that this is really difficult, but I believe in you – I know that you can keep going. It's really important for you to stick with it.*). Brief reminders of the rationale may help, but that can come at the cost of getting started or can distract from the exposure, so they should be limited.
Reducing/stopping safety behaviors	Provide feedback to the patient about safety behaviors that you observe and support them in reducing/stopping those behaviors.	The patient is terrified to stop the safety behavior, and the behavior reduces learning for the patient.	Observe and describe what you notice (*I'm noticing that you keep looking around you, almost as though you are checking who is near you*). Coach the patient to reduce/stop the safety behavior (*I'm wondering if we can practice engaging in the exposure as though you're not nervous, even though I know you are. Practice acting 'as if' you don't need to keep checking to see who is around. Can we try that?*).

continued on next page

Table 4. Continued

Topic	Goal	Challenges	Tips
Modulating emotional intensity	Support the patient in getting emotionally activated or regulated, as needed.	The patient has difficulty with getting in touch with the anxiety during the exposure or experiences such intense emotions that they cannot take in new information to promote learning.	For patients who are experiencing low emotional intensity, help them with staying in the present moment and reducing distraction, and ask them to narrate what they are doing, why, what they are worried will happen as a result. For patients who are experiencing extremely high emotional intensity, ask them to describe what they feel in their body, what is going through their mind, and coach them to observe these intense emotions as they stick with the practice.
Celebrate the wins	Praise as many aspects of the experience as possible, including getting started, sticking with it, and completing the task (as relevant).	Some patients experience shame reactions to praise, which can cause the therapist to reduce the likelihood of providing the necessary praise to celebrate the patient's success.	If praise is genuine, pour it on. Watch videos of yourself providing praise to patients to gauge whether it matched the intensity of praise that you intended. Even when patients are reluctant to sit with praise, gently remind them why it's extremely important to celebrate their successes so that they may find the energy to keep going.
Consolidating the learning after the exposure	Discuss the exposure to highlight new learning.	Rushing, given the limited session time remaining; overemphasis on SUDs reduction as the goal of exposure; post-hoc hypotheses about the exposure being easier than anticipated ("I knew this wouldn't be hard").	Ensure that the exposure will end with sufficient time to discuss the practice and what was learned, and also to plan for ongoing practice. Emphasize whether the feared outcome that was identified prior to the exposure occurred. Return to what was written down *before* the exposure to highlight expectation violation. When the feared outcome occurs, process how the patient's strength allowed them to get through that difficult exposure practice.

- *Point out post-hoc hypotheses:* Often, patients will complete an exposure and report that they did not learn anything from it because they knew it would be easy all along. This post-hoc hypothesis occurs even for exposures that the patient rated as higher on the hierarchy in terms of anticipated SUDs. When the therapist has written down the hypothesis before the exposure, they can reflect this inconsistency back to the patient. For instance:

  It's fascinating because last week, when you were gearing up to do this exposure, you rated the practice as an 80 on the hierarchy, and you told me you were worried that you were going to get so anxious that you would not be able to get anything done at work all week. My memory is that you seemed understandably concerned about it before you left the session. Now that you've done it, you're telling me that you knew it would be easy all along. What do you make of that?

Sometimes it is helpful for patients to know that these post-hoc hypotheses are common, but that they can be discouraging. This is another self-defeating tendency that should be made explicit to the patient and normalized, but not used to dictate major changes to the treatment plan. Rather than downplaying the accomplishment, use this as a "win" to motivate the next steps for exposure practice.

Planning Subsequent *in Vivo* Exposure Practices

After the first *in vivo* exposure exercise is completed, the hierarchy can be used as a tentative treatment plan to guide subsequent practices. Early exposure therapy approaches emphasized "working the way up the hierarchy gradually," and yet research supports the idea that it is not necessary to approach the hierarchy rigidly (Kircanski et al., 2012). As with the first exposure, it is easier to build on your patient's idea for an exposure than it is to convince the patient to try something new. For that reason, a flexible approach toward exposure is recommended. Flexibility in exposure practice can be achieved by following the patient's lead, reducing preoccupation with SUDs as the guiding principle for exposures, and taking "gifts from the universe" in exposure practice. Each of these topics is described in more details below.

Following the Patient's Lead

Therapists have an opportunity to convey their confidence in a patient by allowing the patient to be in the driver's seat in terms of the speed and content of exposure practice. When the patient has had a successful exposure practice, motivation is often high. This is a time to inquire, "In terms of the next *in vivo* practice, what do you think you need to learn next?" The patient may opt to return to their hierarchy to guide the path forward, or they may come up with a new exposure practice altogether. Remember that the hierarchy is a brainstormed list, not a treatment contract. Deviation from the hierarchy is encouraged when the patient has an idea that is intrinsically motivating and objectively safe (by the patient's determination, with evidence from the social network as needed).

Gifts From the Universe

When planning *in vivo* exposures, best practices recommend warning the patient against jumping too far up the hierarchy too soon (Foa et al., 2019). These recommendations are in place to prevent patients from biting off more than they can chew for an exposure, getting discouraged, and dropping out of therapy. Some patients with PTSD will indeed move quickly up the hierarchy and then become overwhelmed, so warning patients to stick to the plan for exposure practices is recommended.

However, sometimes patients encounter a situation that they never might have predicted and that might not present itself in the future. In these situations, we often encourage patients to take these "gift from the universe" exposure practices as rare opportunities to learn about their capacity to tolerate anxiety. Given the principles of inhibitory learning, unexpected exposure practices can promote expectation violation. When patients come to session with a gift from the universe exposure, praise their bravery for jumping at a chance to push themselves. Consider also using this as an opportunity to evaluate what the impact of the exposure was on their motivation for treatment. Some patients may feel discouraged after trying to do something that was too challenging too quickly (as discussed earlier in this chapter). In those cases, therapists praise the effort rather than the outcome. Other patients may feel a renewed resolution in the treatment plan, in which case praising the effort and the outcome is warranted.

Conducting *in Vivo* Exposures With the Patient

While nearly all CBT approaches for PTSD emphasize *in vivo* exposure practices, manuals differ in terms of whether the therapist should accompany the patient on their first or a subsequent *in vivo* exposure. In PE, *in vivo* exposure practices are assigned in session 2 for completion independently (i.e., without the therapist) before session 3. In contrast, in the Unified Protocol, the therapist usually accompanies the patient on their first *in vivo* exposure exercise and in-session exposures are recommended initially wherever possible (Barlow, Farchione, et al., 2017). There are pros and cons to both approaches (see Table 5).

Table 5. Pros and cons of therapist-accompanied *in vivo* exposure practices

Situation	Pro	Con
In vivo exposures conducted without the therapist	The patient increases their sense of accomplishment and feels capable of future independent practice.	The therapist misses an opportunity to observe how the patient is completing the practice, including paying attention to the use of safety behaviors or other avoidance strategies, and to encourage the patient to stay in the present moment and see the exposure through until the end.
In vivo exposures conducted with the therapist	The therapist has an opportunity to encourage the patient to stay in the present moment, see the exposure through until the end, and to drop safety behaviors. The therapist can adjust the plans for the exposure as needed to promote optimal learning.	The patient may have a harder time initiating exposures on their own in the future.
In vivo exposures initially conducted independently unless a problem arises	This balanced approach allows the patient to feel more independent in their *in vivo* exposure practice, but to eventually get the support that they need to optimize learning in future practices (especially for more challenging exposures).	If early independent exposures are discouraging to the patient, the patient is at greater risk of dropping out or feeling unmotivated for more exposure practices. Even when the therapist joins a subsequent exposure, the patient may have already decided that the approach is too difficult or unhelpful.

Regardless of whether the patient and therapist decide on independent or partnered *in vivo* exposure exercises, there is a need for flexibility based on how the practices unfold. The goal of the exposure is to promote optimal learning, and the patient and therapist should prioritize this goal when selecting their approach.

Summary

For patients with PTSD, *in vivo* exposures offer opportunities for new learning about their anxiety, empowerment, threat from others, and ability to function even in the face of high-intensity emotions. *In vivo* exposures should be introduced with a strong psychoeducation and rationale to justify the treatment approach. Next, patient and therapist should collaboratively generate a list of activities that the patient can practice approaching, rather than avoiding, which are rated for difficulty using a SUDs rating. Then, patients generate their expectations for each exposure and begin to practice the exercises repeatedly. When patients struggle to complete exposure practices, they may benefit from discussions to increase their willingness to practice in the future. Patients' learning is maximized by discussing whether expectation violation occurred.

6 Optimizing Imaginal Exposure

Imaginal exposure is akin to a process of storytelling, long recognized as a therapeutic tradition across many cultures (Brave Heart & DeBruyn, 1998; Briant et al., 2016; Chioneso et al., 2020; East et al., 2010). In some gold-standard therapies for PTSD, such as PE therapy (Foa et al., 2007, 2019), imaginal exposure is introduced early in treatment (as early as session 3) and dominates most in-session therapy content. In fact, some research has compared the relative importance of imaginal or *in vivo* exposure homework and found that higher adherence to imaginal exposure homework predicted improved therapy outcomes for PTSD, whereas adherence to *in vivo* exposure homework was unrelated to therapy outcomes (Cooper et al., 2017). For this reason, imaginal exposure is a highly recommended therapeutic component when treating PTSD.

How to Introduce Imaginal Exposure to Patients With PTSD

Many clinicians are often reluctant to engage in imaginal exposure (Ross et al., 2022; Whiteside, 2023), even though patients typically report that they would like to use exposure for treatment of PTSD (Becker et al., 2007). While *in vivo* exposures are often difficult for patients at first, many patients are terrified at the prospect of telling the story of their trauma. Patients often report that they are "hanging on by a thread" at the point when they get to therapy and have little confidence in their own ability to manage and tolerate the strong negative emotions that imaginal exposure may provoke. These negative cognitions about the self are sometimes (inadvertently) reinforced by loved ones who are worried about the patient pushing themselves to discuss painful things. In some cases, even other clinicians might have actively discouraged the patient from discussing their trauma. For these reasons, it is not uncommon for patients to present for therapy feeling very reluctant to talk about their trauma in any level of detail. Below are some strategies for managing this reluctance while supporting the client's autonomy to make a decision that works best for them.

Normalizing Reluctance to Discuss the Trauma

In most initial evaluations for PTSD, I leave about 15 minutes to describe the therapeutic approach and rationale. After hearing this brief overview, patients commonly express some reservations about imaginal exposures. Many patients have said, "I've spent years trying not to think about the trauma, and now you want me to talk about it?" After many years of doing this work in clinical and research settings, I can confidently reassure patients that their anticipatory anxiety about discussing the trauma is a strong indication that we are planning the correct treatment approach. I often say to patients, *If you weren't expressing some reluctance to talk about the trauma, I would probably be thinking that we might not need to do this. Your reaction is common – almost everyone with whom I've done this therapy has some version of this reaction. In fact, not wanting to talk about the trauma is one of the hallmark symptoms of PTSD. Your reaction also tells me that this is exactly how we should proceed, if you are willing.*

Using Metaphor to Build Buy-in for Imaginal Exposures

I often use numerous metaphors drawn from PE therapy (Foa et al., 2007, 2019) or acceptance and commitment therapy (Hayes et al., 1999) to help build buy-in for imaginal exposure. One of my favorite metaphors comes from the PE manual (Foa et al., 2007, 2019), wherein imaginal exposure serves many core functions, including improving the context surrounding the memory and helping the patient to emotionally process it. To highlight this point, the PE manual describes a trauma memory as similar to picking up a book, reading a line on a page, having a negative reaction to the line, and slamming the book closed. Similarly, patients with PTSD will experience intrusive memories about their trauma and immediately attempt to suppress the memory or distract from it. The PE manual (Foa et al., 2007, 2019) describes that imaginal exposure is similar to picking the book up and reading the full chapter, giving the sentence context, and helping the patient to emotionally process the content of the chapter. As discussed in Chapter 9, dealing with negative cognitions, a trauma memory without context reinforces negative cognitions about the self and the world. For instance, an assault survivor might have an intrusive memory of being overpowered during the attack and think, "Why didn't I fight back more?" In telling the full story of the trauma, the survivor has the opportunity to remember the context of why they reacted as they did and to begin the healing process. Note, though, that usually these contextual revelations are hard for patients to believe until they experience them – early in treatment, you will not be able to convince the patient that talking through the trauma will give them context that they currently do not have. Indeed, they lived through the trauma and the therapist did not, so the patient has intimate knowledge of their experience that the therapist should not downplay. They are the expert on their own experiences, and the therapist is in a role of supportive coach to facilitate their working through the most difficult chapter or chapters in their history. Nevertheless, I find that the chapter metaphor resonates with many patients as it demonstrates a need to emotionally digest the trauma.

Other patients agree with the concept of imaginal exposure but are very fearful about what emotional reactions the procedure might evoke in them. For this concern, I commonly draw on a metaphor from acceptance and commitment therapy (Hayes et al., 1999), likening imaginal exposure to cleaning an old coffee mug with stuck-on coffee grounds (or in my family, oatmeal bowls that my husband and daughter left in the sink). To get the mug clean, you must fill it with water and soapy suds, and the grounds get all mixed into a mushy mess before they finally get unstuck. Imaginal exposure similarly can involve emotionally messy work in the service of cleaning out the internal wounds of trauma.

Distinguishing Imaginal Exposure From Casual Discussions About the Trauma

Some patients with PTSD have had to talk about their trauma repeatedly, whether because of police investigations, custody battles, evaluations for disability, or other legal reasons. These patients may understandably wonder how more discussions about their trauma could possibly help. As discussed in PE (Foa et al., 2007, 2019), imaginal exposure is distinct from police report versions of trauma discussions, in which the patient shares a version of the necessary details about the trauma but often forgoes emotional connection to its meaning (or intentionally suppresses that emotional provocation for many legitimate reasons). In imaginal exposure, the patient is encouraged to discuss the memories while allowing themselves to feel whatever they need to feel to promote healing.

Freedom of Choice and Absence of Alternatives

It is my belief (without any studies to directly support this view) that, like all therapeutic techniques, imaginal exposure will not work for people who are not willing to engage in it. Naturally, there is no way to ethically evaluate this hypothesis, as we cannot force people to do imaginal exposures if they are unwilling. Regardless, the therapist's role is to provide patients with new strategies to try for managing or treating their PTSD, without trying to convince or coerce them. In dialectical behavior therapy (Linehan, 1993), patients are introduced to the concept of "freedom of choice, absence of alternatives." In other words, the patient must retain the freedom to choose whether to engage in imaginal exposure. If they opt not to engage in this procedure, there may not be ideal alternatives. Certainly, many studies have demonstrated that other nonexposure therapy options, especially CPT (Resick et al., 2016), have a strong evidence base and do not include imaginal exposure. However, therapies that retain imaginal exposure as a core component, especially PE, have the strongest evidence base for recommendations according to multiple meta-analyses (Cusack et al., 2016; Powers et al., 2010) and clinical practice guidelines (American Psychological Association, 2017; VA/DoD, 2023). When a patient is unwilling to conduct imaginal exposure, I will educate them about CPT and provide them with referrals to other therapists. However, I also express concern that their trauma memory might continue to haunt them if they do not spend the time to process the memory sufficiently. I always encourage getting second opinions from other experts and invite patients to take some time to think it over. Almost always, this pressure-free approach results in a patient's decision to proceed with imaginal exposure.

Imaginal Exposure Practice

The First Imaginal Exposure Practice

In PE, imaginal exposure begins on session 3, but the patient starts preparing for it as early as session 1. During session 1 in PE, the patient and therapist collaboratively agree on start and end points for the imaginal exposures during the trauma history interview, an interview that is conducted to gather contextual information about the trauma. By gathering the start and end points of the trauma memory before session 3, the therapist saves some time, allowing for greater rapidity when jumping into imaginal exposures in session. This offers a great advantage when patients (and clinicians) have anticipatory anxiety about imaginal exposures and are tempted to delay getting started.

However, the downside of collecting these start and end points in session 1 is that to gather this information, the patient needs to start talking about their trauma. Even with instructions to share only a few details about the trauma (just enough to know where to start and end), patients sometimes divulge the full details of it. This leads to an awkward exchange – the patient has accidentally started doing an imaginal exposure without the proper coaching on how to do it, and without the proper buy-in about why they are doing it. The elicitation of start and end points also invites an opportunity for the therapist to have to "correct" the patient when they start telling too many details about the trauma and need to be interrupted. This correction may reinforce the patient's own beliefs that they are not ready to discuss their trauma. Even when navigated skillfully and conscientiously, it may also slightly damage rapport. Finally, gathering start and end points for the imaginal exposure in session 1 builds even more anticipatory anxiety for patients when they begin imaginal exposures in a subsequent session because it may stir up some emotional distress that the patients have been instructed to bottle up in order to return to the trauma in a future session. Countless clinical trials have been conducted following Foa and colleagues' (2007, 2019) procedure of identifying start and end points in session 1 and have shown strong improvements in PTSD symptoms, but you may need to approach this thoughtfully for the reasons described here.

Regardless of when the start and end points are gathered, imaginal exposure is conducted based on a "slice of time." The process involves retelling the trauma as though it were happening again (in first person, present tense) from the beginning to the end, and then repeating the story multiple times in each session. In PE, imaginal exposures were originally designed to last 45–60 minutes, but a recent noninferiority study determined that 20 minutes of imaginal exposure performed comparably to 40 minutes (Foa et al., 2022). In the Unified Protocol (Barlow, Sauer-Zavala, et al., 2017), there is no time-based recommendation for sticking with the exposure practice. Thus, the timing of the imaginal exposure is likely not as important as the patient having multiple opportunities to sit with the memory of what happened to invite healing.

In PE and the Unified Protocol for PTSD, imaginal exposure is often recommended with the patient closing their eyes and retelling the story of what happened to them. The story should include sensory details, cognitions that the patient had during the trauma, and emotional reactions that the patient had during the trauma, in addition to the play-by-play of what happened during the event. Ideally, patients are coached to tell the story in the first person and the present tense, but these instructions are not meant to be rigidly followed, especially in the first imaginal exposure. When the patient comes to the end of the story, they are asked to return to the beginning and repeat the story until the time for imaginal exposure practice is over. The imaginal exposure should also be recorded to allow for homework completion.

For the first imaginal exposure, I typically recommend that the therapist asks for what they want to see and then praises whatever they get, without much correction. The number one objective for the first imaginal exposure is coaching the patient to tell the story of what happened to them; the number two objective is to keep the patient "in the boat" of therapy. This means that the therapist must toe the line between boosting patients' confidence in their ability to tell the story and not pushing them too far, too fast. Especially in the first imaginal exposure, the therapist should make it clear that the patient is in control.

Therapist Behavior During Imaginal Exposure Practice

After the therapist provides the instructions for how to do the imaginal exposure, they have a few key tasks, with core objectives tied to those tasks, and common mistakes that new (and experienced) therapists make related to these tasks (see Table 6). These tasks include serving as support provider, timekeeper, hypothesis generator, outside observer, distress monitor, and clarifier. Across all tasks, it is critical to balance providing support with staying out of the patient's way. A therapist who is too quiet runs the risk of the patient feeling alone in their painful recollection of the trauma, but a therapist who is too active interrupts the process and reduces the patient's confidence. The best way to gauge whether the therapist is sufficiently active is for the therapist to video-record the session and watch themselves.

In their role as outside observer and hypothesis generator, the therapist should attend to nonverbal and verbal cues about the source of what is preventing emotional healing in the patient. Rather than verbally noting these observations, the therapist should write them down to ask the patient about after the imaginal exposure. If the therapist thinks that they have a question to ask during the imaginal exposure, they should first consider whether the question is necessary at that moment. In most cases, questions can (and should) be held until after the imaginal exposure is over to allow the patient to get into a flow as they tell their story. The "staying out of the way" advice is most important during the first imaginal exposure, when the patient feels most vulnerable in telling their story.

Approximately every 5 minutes, the therapist should assess the patient's distress using SUDs (see Chapter 5). This assessment should be conducted in an unobtrusive manner by agreeing on a brief query that the therapist will verbalize, such as "SUDs?" or "Level?" Patients are often confused about whether the the therapist is asking about the SUDs experienced now (in the therapy office) or then (during the trauma). The therapist is indeed inquiring about distress *now*, which is confusing. For this reason, it is important to not get obsessive about the SUDs levels and to request that the patient just go with their gut reaction rather than overthinking it.

Table 6. Tasks during imaginal exposure

Task	Objective	Common Therapist Mistakes
Support the patient	Use verbal communication to remind the patient of your presence and your confidence in them.	The therapist feels high anxiety about the patient being upset, resulting in too frequent communications of support that distract the patient.
Timekeeper	Write down the start time of the imaginal exposure, the anticipated end time, and write out every 5 minutes in between as times to assess the patient's subjective units of distress (SUDs). Calmly invite the patient to open their eyes after the last repetition.	The therapist loses track of time, and the session runs over. The therapist is anxious about the imaginal exposure being too upsetting and ends it early.
Hypothesis generator	Take detailed notes while the patient recounts the story, with particular attention to trying to uncover trauma-related negative cognitions that are preventing healing.	The therapist assumes that the source of what is "keeping the patient stuck" should be obvious in the first few sessions.
Outside observer	Observe the patients' body language, emotional upset, and word choices to gather an outsider's perspective on how the trauma is affecting the patient.	The therapist points these details out to the patient too early (before sufficient rapport has been built) in an attempt to speed up the process.
Distress monitor	Prompt for SUDs approximately every 5 minutes.	The therapist asks too frequently or not frequently enough; only assessing between repetitions.
Clarifier	Ask *brief* questions to clarify the details of the story, the emotional reaction, core cognitions for the patient (during the trauma itself), physical sensations about the trauma.	The therapist is too distracting; asking too many, lengthy, or unnecessary questions.

Second Imaginal Exposure Practice

Before the second imaginal exposure begins, the therapist has a window of opportunity to praise the patient's prior work and to model a different strategy to use for the next dose. For some patients, the recommendation is to slow down, and the therapist can model the ideal pacing. For other patients, the recommendation is about removing "breaks" (where the patient is engaging in avoidance behaviors to reduce their emotional intensity) and the therapist should model how to speak fluidly without excessive pauses. This corrective feedback can always be framed as *I was thinking a lot about your bravery last time and you did such an amazing job with the exposure. I'm really proud of you. This time, I want us to try it a little differently. I think it would be helpful if you...* [enter feedback, with a focus on only one constructive change]. *Would you be willing to give that a try this time?* Even when patients consent to changing how they do the practice, it can be difficult for them to break the habit of how they do the imaginal exposure because sometimes these strategies are mostly about reducing their distress (in other words, they are not accidental).

Subsequent Imaginal Exposures

As patients become more accustomed to engaging in imaginal exposures, it becomes possible to increase the use of targeted questions as needed. Questions should be kept brief, and only asked when the patient:

- Is glossing over important parts of the memory
- Is not providing enough of a story to form a mental image of the scene in the therapist's imagination
- Is not describing a core component of the memory (no mention of emotions, cognitions, or sensations)
- Seems to get stuck at a part of the memory with each repetition

As imaginal exposures progress, it is common for therapists to coach patients to shorten the length of the imaginal exposure by narrowing the start and end points. In PE therapy (Foa et al., 2007, 2019), this reduction in the length of the imaginal exposure is formally referred to as "hot spots," which are usually 2–4 minutes of content that the patient has the opportunity to repeat many more times in a single session. The selection of hot spots is based on the part of the memory that the patient reports is the most difficult part, and there may be more than one for a patient. In PE, hot spots are usually introduced between sessions 6 and 9. In other variants of CBT, the imaginal exposure length may be shortened without using a formal hot spot truncation. Common patterns include the following:

- High activation one session, low activation the next: Patients who become extremely upset during one imaginal exposure session often come to the following session with a "shut-down" presentation. These patients are sometimes engaging in active strategies to numb themselves from the memory so that they do not become too upset during the exposure.
- Stable SUDs: We often gauge the overall success of treatment if the peak SUDs rating (the highest SUDs in each imaginal exposure session) is trending downward. This does not always occur and, as discussed in Chapter 5, treatment can still be successful even if SUDs remain high during imaginal exposures.
- Homework: For each session, the patient will have a new recording of their imaginal exposure that they can listen to for homework. As part of CBT for PTSD, I usually ask the patient to listen to the recording at least three times between sessions, whereas PE usually assigns daily practice. As with everything else in this book, ask for what you want to see and praise whatever you get.

Summary

Imaginal exposures are a very important aspect of CBT for PTSD. These exposures allow the patient to discuss the story of their trauma in a safe and nonjudgmental atmosphere. Patients and therapists alike are often trepidatious about imaginal exposures before they experience the process. Once both parties gain experience with this component of CBT for PTSD, many find that it is a core driver of improvement for patients with PTSD.

7 Optimizing Interoceptive Exposures

Exposure therapy for PTSD focuses on a combination of imaginal and *in vivo* exposure exercises. However, some patients report extremely high interoceptive sensitivity, which can disrupt the treatment process. For these patients, it may be helpful to introduce them to *interoceptive exposure*, or exposure to feared bodily sensations.

Rationale for Interoceptive Exposure Practice

Some patients with PTSD report significant fears about the consequences of feeling strong physical sensations. Like patients with panic disorder, some patients with PTSD worry that if they feel strong physical sensations, they might lose control or "do something crazy." These individuals cope with fears of physical sensations by attempting to suppress them, which, in turn, backfires and increases anxiety. Drawing on research among patients with panic disorder (Lee et al., 2006), some patients with PTSD may demonstrate a predictable cognitive model underlying fears of physical sensations (see Figure 2).

Like patients with panic disorder, an individual who starts to fear physical sensations in the face of trauma-related reminders might increase avoidance of those reminders even further. They might also begin to increase self-monitoring of the presence/absence of uncomfortable physical sensations. The more an individual with PTSD looks for evidence that their body is betraying them, the more likely they are to find evidence supporting this belief. Then, when those sensations are detected, a person with PTSD might respond by attempting to suppress those sensations through further avoidance strategies. In the short run, avoidance may reduce physical sensations, but in the long run, avoidance increases those sensations, completing the self-perpetuating cycle. Given this cycle (monitoring → noticing physical sensations → avoidance → monitoring...), an individual with PTSD must create opportunities to feel these uncomfortable physical sensations without avoiding them to learn about their relative danger/safety. Interoceptive exposures offer an opportunity to promote such learning.

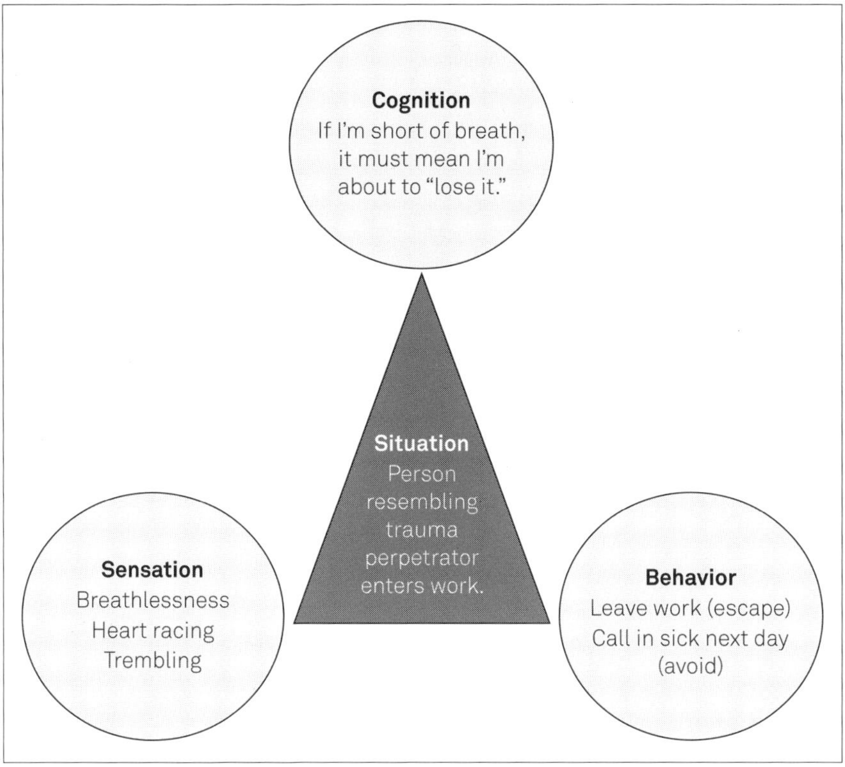

Figure 2. Cognitive model of interoceptive sensitivity among patients with PTSD.

As with all exposures, the goal of interoceptive exposures is to create a new inhibitory association, wherein physical sensations become paired with the perception of safety, rather than the excitatory association, wherein they are paired with the perception of danger. Over time, interoceptive exposures work to retrain the brain and reduce false alarms about low-grade physical sensations. For patients with PTSD who are very bothered by physical sensations in the context of trauma reminders, these exposures can be key to improving self-confidence.

Information Gathering for Interoceptive Exposures

Following protocols from CBT for panic disorder (Craske et al., 2007), interoceptive exposures are always preceded by a data gathering exercise, the goal for which is to determine which exercises provoke high distress (SUDs) or provoke sensations that closely resemble the uncomfortable sensations when encountering a trauma reminder. The therapist should explain the exercise to the patient and then elicit the patient's feared expectation for the exercise (see Handout 4). In other words, after the patient understands what they are being asked to do, what are they most worried will occur because of the interoceptive exposure? As with all exposure practices, elicitation of the expectation before the information-gathering activity allows for more opportunity to promote inhibitory learning through highlighting expectation violation (if such occurs). Even if patients do not have feared expectations for a particular exercise, it can still be helpful to attempt the exposure for the purposes of information gathering. Because we tend to do a poor job of predicting the future, some interoceptive exposures may be more difficult than expected and others may be less difficult. Difficulty also depends upon the patient's baseline anxiety at the start of the practice or other vulnerability factors (e.g., whether the patient got sufficient sleep the night before, had enough to eat for breakfast, or had too much coffee that day).

The therapist should engage in the exercises with the patient to both increase the patient's confidence in the safety of the activity and to reduce their self-consciousness about the exercises. Typically, the therapist and patient will begin the exercise with a stopwatch to track timing closely, and the patient is asked to raise their hand or otherwise communicate when they notice upsetting sensations. Once the patient raises their hand, the therapist usually asks the patient to continue for another 10–15 seconds. Then, the patient rates their SUDs and resemblance of the sensations to an upsetting panic attack. For information-gathering purposes, the therapist and patient then take a brief break before shifting to the next exercise. These activities can stir up distress, quickly in some patients (in as short a time as 10 seconds), whereas for others, it takes time for the anxiety to build (90 seconds to 2 minutes). If the exercise does not elicit any distress, the therapist and patient can shift to the next exercise after 90 seconds to 2 minutes. As this information-gathering phase is conducted exclusively for the purpose of building a symptom hierarchy, habituation of distress is not an explicit goal of the activities. However, it can be helpful to track the patient's recovery time (i.e., how long it took for SUDs to decrease after each exercise) as part of information gathering. Most importantly, by engaging in these exercises with the patient, the goal is to demystify physical sensations and coach the patient toward becoming their own scientist about their physical experiences.

Types of Interoceptive Exposure Practices

There are a multitude of common interoceptive exposure practices conducted in CBT for panic disorder that can be useful for treating PTSD. Listed below are four common exercises to begin information gathering. If your patient has other ideas for activities to complete that stir up physical sensations, be sure to follow their lead.

Hyperventilation

Our research has demonstrated that in a transdiagnostic sample, disrupted breathing is the most common symptom of panic attacks regardless of the principal diagnosis (Brown et al., 2016). This is likely attributable to the close connection between the ratio of carbon dioxide/oxygen and anxiety provocation outside of panic attacks (Meuret et al., 2011). Given the prevalence of disrupted breathing as a core panic attack symptom, hyperventilation interoceptive exposure exercises usually trigger significant SUDs scores or elicit sensations that closely resemble panic attack sensations occurring in the context of trauma triggers (or otherwise). To engage in this practice, the therapist and patient quickly and repeatedly take deep in-breaths of air with very short exhales.

Spinning

When patients are fearful of physical sensations, dizziness can be extremely disconcerting. Spinning interoceptive exercises can be conducted in a chair that spins (usually this is easier) or by standing and spinning (usually this is harder).

Derealization

This exercise is accomplished by holding a handheld mirror up to the patient's face and having the patient stare directly into their own eyes. This exercise tends to be polarizing – for many patients, it elicits no sensations whatsoever, but for a select few, it is extremely unnerving and closely mimics the derealization symptoms that occur during panic attacks.

Physical Exercise

Any form of physical exercise can cause distress for a patient with PTSD who is fearful of their bodily sensations. Commonly conducted exercises include burpees, jumping jacks, or running in place.

Assigning Interoceptive Exposure Practices

The First Interoceptive Exposure Practice

After determining which types of exercises are difficult for the patient, it can be helpful to take a systematic approach toward assigning interoceptive practice. Usually, two types of exercises are assigned. For some patients, SUDs decrease quickly during these practice exercises, and this more commonly occurs when patients push themselves to complete many repetitions of the exercises, especially in varied contexts (internal and external). For this reason, it can be helpful to assign brief bursts of these exercises. You might suggest that the patient practice exercise A three times in a row, with a brief break in between, and to repeat this practice three times daily between sessions. Assigning an alternative exercise (practice exercise B) can be useful when the patient experiences a quick reduction in distress about practice exercise A, and it can help the patient boost their confidence because it increases the difficulty level. As with everything in CBT for PTSD, the goal is to ask for what you want to see and then praise whatever you get.

After praising any homework completion, the goal is to promote inhibitory learning by highlighting expectation violation. Given that the exercises were preceded by elicitation of feared expectations, the therapist should inquire about whether a feared expectation occurred during any of the practice exposures. If the feared outcome *did* occur when the patient was engaging in the interoceptive exposure practice, the therapist can inquire about how they got through the very difficult practice to highlight the patient's strength and resilience. In all other circumstances, the therapist can inquire about the patient's interpretation of the expectation violation. In other words, what did it mean to the patient that the feared outcome did not occur? What does that say about the physical sensations, the patient's competence, or the patient's emotion regulation capacity?

Subsequent Interoceptive Exposure Practices

Once the patient has completed their first interoceptive exposure practice, they can mix up the practice exercises or go in the order of difficulty, depending on the patient's preference. As described above, some exercises will be relatively more or less difficult when the patient is in a different emotional state before an exercise or has different vulnerability factors. It is essential to remind the patient that they are in charge of the pacing of practice exercises and that you will support them with their decisions about how to progress. In the service of demystifying the exercise, it is helpful to model a scientific approach where the decision about which exposure practice to engage in is based on what the patient needs to learn about themselves.

Summary

Some patients with PTSD report high interoceptive sensitivity and may benefit from interoceptive exposure to internal cues. The goal of interoceptive exposure is to learn that physical sensations are not dangerous. This can be achieved by intentionally provoking the sensation and learning to sit with it, without changing behavior to avoid the sensation. Over time, patients learn that these sensations are not dangerous and increase their confidence that they can tolerate them.

8 Behavioral Activation

As described in Chapter 1, PTSD is highly comorbid with major depressive disorder (MDD; Brown, Jerud, et al., 2018). Up to 52% of patients with PTSD have a concurrent diagnosis of MDD (Rytwinski et al., 2013). Patients with PTSD who report anhedonia (a core symptom of MDD) exhibit notable deficits in reward processing in a manner that is similar to patients with MDD (Nawijn et al., 2015). This deficit might result in potentially rewarding activities not being experienced as such among patients with PTSD and anhedonia. Thus, therapists must carefully attend to this comorbidity as part of their treatment planning.

My prior research, drawing on data from multiple studies of prolonged exposure (PE; $N = 216$), demonstrated that there was a reciprocal relationship between depression and PTSD symptoms in PE (Brown, Jerud, et al., 2018). In other words, patients' PTSD symptom severity during a given session predicted their depression symptom severity in the subsequent session, and vice versa. In cognitive processing therapy (CPT), the largest study to date on this topic demonstrated that PTSD and depression changed concurrently in treatment (Liverant et al., 2012). These findings suggest that for a patient with significant PTSD and depression symptoms, evidence-based PTSD treatments will likely improve secondary depression, and that when depression improves, PTSD symptoms improve as well. Thus, there is value in exploring strategies to gain momentum in reducing depression among patients with PTSD. Behavioral activation and pleasant event scheduling is one of the most reliable therapeutic interventions to improve depression.

Data Gathering

In traditional CBT for depression, behavioral activation begins by gathering data on the relationship between activities, accomplishment, and pleasure. Specifically, patients usually spend one week mapping out how they spend their waking hours and tracking accomplishment (on a 0–10-point Likert scale, where 0 is no sense of accomplishment and 10 is extremely accomplished), pleasure (on a 0–10-point Likert scale, where 0 is the least enjoyable and 10 is the most enjoyable a task could be), and sometimes overall mood (on a 0–10-point Likert scale, where 0 is the worst it could ever be and 10 is the best it could ever be; Kanter et al., 2010). To track these data, patients can use one of myriad worksheets available for free online, a mood tracker mobile app, a simple piece of paper that they design based on their preference, or a notes app on their phone.

After patients have gathered data on their activities, accomplishment, pleasure, and mood, these data should be reviewed collaboratively to detect notable patterns. It is helpful to observe whether there are activities that reliably increase accomplishment in the absence of pleasure and vice versa, as well as activities that have high or low scores on both accomplishment and pleasure. Patients commonly observe that, even in their free time, they spent multiple hours during the week on activities that are associated with low accomplishment and low pleasure. Common examples of nonreinforcing (but high-likelihood) behaviors include binge-watching television or mindlessly scrolling through social media. Patients may notice that these behaviors are occasionally relaxing or enjoyable, but the pleasure derived from such activities is not reliable. These high-likelihood behaviors are rarely associated with a sense of accomplishment. Alternatively, patients often observe that activities focused on self-care and completing chores can increase a sense of accomplishment even if they are not enjoyable. A third common tendency is for patients to observe that they procrastinated on doing a task earlier in the week but that, when completed, the task was associated with a major sense of accomplishment. Each of these observations is a critical source of data that can be useful to inspire intervention opportunities.

Brainstorming Activities to Boost Accomplishment or Pleasure

After the patient and therapist discover core patterns of associations among activities and accomplishment, pleasure, and mood, the next step is to generate a list of activities that have a chance of increasing either accomplishment or pleasure or both. This list can include:

- Activities that the patient rated as high accomplishment or pleasure from their data-gathering phase
- Activities that the patient used to enjoy, even if they no longer do them
- Activities from which the patient used to derive a sense of accomplishment, even if they no longer do them
- Activities that the patient hypothesizes might be experienced as enjoyable or self-esteem boosting, even if they have never tried them

- Activities that other people have wanted the patient to do and that have a chance of being enjoyable/accomplishment boosting
- Activities from well-published lists of "pleasant events," which are easy to access with a quick internet search

Much like when the *in vivo* hierarchy list is generated for the first time, the activities list that the patient generates does not have to be perfect the first time. This list should be conceptualized as a jumping-off point for potential behavioral activation items to come. Given that PTSD often results in a narrowing of activities for individuals, I often frame this brainstorming exercise to patients as generating a list of activities to grow their lives in meaningful directions. Sometimes it is also helpful to frame these activities as things that patients could do to treat themselves or to be kind to themselves.

Behavioral Activation Practice

Agreeing on the First Behavioral Activation Practice

As with selecting the first *in vivo* exposure exercise, it is ideal when the patient feels supported to choose their behavioral activation items rather than having items assigned to them. When the patient is having a difficult time selecting their first behavioral activation item, they can be reminded that this is an experimental process, and it is totally acceptable to try an activity even if they are not sure that it will be enjoyable. It might help to narrow the list to three possibilities to reduce decision fatigue for the patient. It might also help to remind them that even if they are tempted to put pressure on themselves to do a lot all at once, it is more helpful to select one small thing to do to build momentum rather than overcommit (and ultimately feel disappointed if they should fail).

Building Commitment

Once the patient identifies that they have an activity that they are willing to complete for behavioral activation practice, it can be helpful to return to the commitment-building exercises discussed earlier (for *in vivo* exposure practices, see Chapter 5). Specifically, consider asking the patient how likely it is that they will complete the behavioral activation activity on a 0–100% scale, where 100% is "This will definitely happen, no doubt about it" and 0% is "I already know that I won't do this." If the patient rates their likelihood of doing the activity as any score less than 80%, there is a high risk of noncompletion.

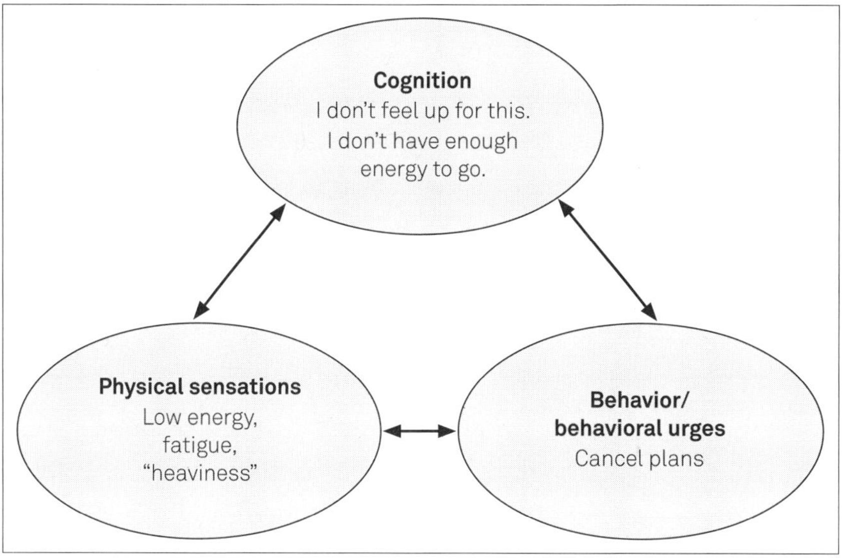

Figure 3. A cognitive model describing a patient who decides to cancel social plans.

In those cases, it may be helpful to proactively change the exercise to make it easier. Even if the patient indicates a high likelihood of doing the activity, it can still be helpful to proactively schedule the activity in their calendar or brainstorm potential obstacles that they might encounter and solutions to those obstacles.

By the time you are collaboratively selecting the patient's first behavioral activation item, you might have already learned about the patient's cognitive behavioral patterns to support them in making a successful plan. For instance, perhaps you have observed your patient engaging in a pattern of making plans with friends but then canceling at the last minute. This patient might report that low energy, not feeling "up for it," fears of judgment from others, or fear of PTSD triggers might drive the behavior of canceling plans. An example cognitive model reflecting this pattern is exhibited in Figure 3.

As is typical in these cognitive and behavioral patterns, the patient might report that when they cancel plans, they immediately feel a sense of relief. The relief is shortly followed by increased loneliness, depression, and listlessness; negative cognitions about the self might increase, as might cognitions about being judged by other people as "flaky" or unreliable.

When you have evidence that your patient has fallen into a cognitive and behavioral trap like the pattern illustrated in Figure 3, it can be helpful to anticipate this pattern reemerging prior to the first behavioral activation exercise. For instance, the therapist might start this conversation as follows:

Therapist: I'm so delighted that you're going to make plans with one of your friends for your behavioral activation activity this week. I know that in the past, there have been times when you attempted to make plans like this with other people and ultimately backed out at the last minute. I know you had some good reasons for doing so at the time –do you remember that?

Patient: Yes, I know exactly what you're talking about because it happens to me all the time.

Therapist: OK, that's helpful to know. Maybe we can use that to our advantage and proactively think this through. What might happen this time that will make it harder for you to stick to the plan of keeping your social plans?

Patient: The biggest thing is just not feeling like it. Sometimes I'm actually looking forward to seeing my friends when I make the plans, but by the time the day comes for the plans, I'm usually so exhausted. Between work and all the stuff I have to do just to get by, sometimes it feels like there is nothing left over. Then I start to think that maybe I just don't have the energy to keep the plans, and I end up bailing.

Therapist: I see, that makes a lot of sense. What happens when you bail?

Patient: Well that's kind of the problem – nothing happens. Usually, my friends are pretty nice and understanding of everything that I'm going through, so most of them don't give me a hard time. They always know there's a chance of me flaking when I make plans with them – sometimes they even joke about it with me, which doesn't

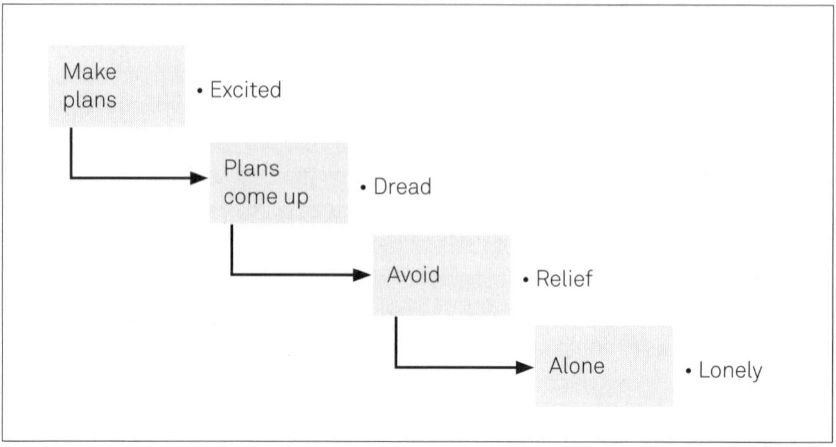

Figure 4. Social plans paradox, Part 1: The trap.

feel great. On the one hand, I'm glad that I'm not disappointing them, but on the other hand, it doesn't make me feel great about myself. I start to feel like a loser.

Therapist: OK, this sounds really important. So your friends don't exactly try to make you feel guilty about canceling plans, but they have also made it clear that they feel they might not be able to rely on you for those social plans. That takes a toll on how you see yourself. Are there any other negative consequences of canceling the plans?

Patient: As ridiculous as this sounds, sometimes I end up feeling way worse at the end of the night. It's like, I'm canceling plans to feel like I'm taking it easier on myself or giving myself a break, but usually I actually feel really bad later in the day. Lonelier and like things are kind of pointless.

Therapist: I'm hearing that things backfire; you are canceling the plans to get more rest, but the rest isn't restful because you feel more isolated. I call this pattern the social plans paradox (see Figure 4). In this paradox, you make plans and even feel excited about them. Then the day of the event comes, and you feel some dread or low energy, which makes you decide to avoid the plans by canceling. When you cancel, you get almost instantaneous relief, but then you are more alone and consequently feel lonelier. Does that sound right to you?

Patient: Yes, that sounds about right. It's basically my life right now.

Therapist: There is an alternative here, of course. I'm guessing you already know what that might be.

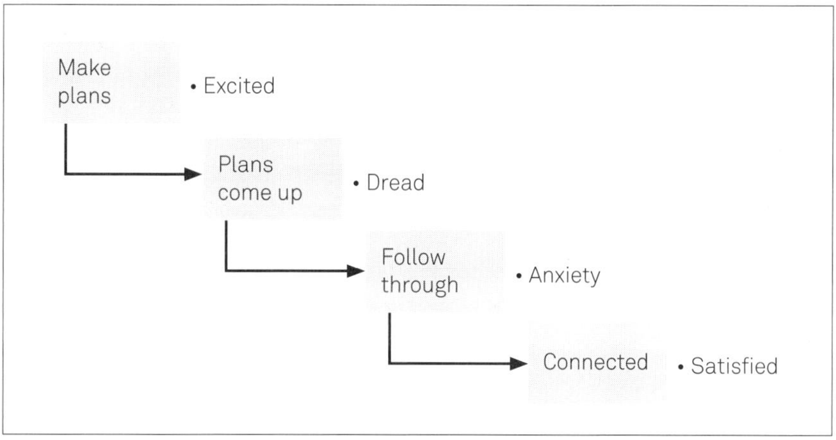

Figure 5. Social plans paradox, Part 2: An alternative solution.

Patient: Probably something like, suck it up and do it . . .

Therapist: Yes, that's basically it. If you hold yourself accountable to your social network and follow through on your plans, rather than canceling, there is this alternative solution that emerges (see Figure 5). In the solution, you follow through on your plans, which might increase anxiety in the short run, but then you end up feeling more connected and more satisfied with your relationships and your life in general. Now I know that's easier said than done, but if you can get yourself to stick to it, there's a good chance that it will help you feel much better, faster. So, the question is: How can we get you to follow through on these plans, even when you might want to cancel?

Patient: That's the million-dollar question! One thing is to tell my friends that I'm legitimately trying to work on this and to ask them to help me. I know that they usually want to help me, but they don't know how. So maybe if I tell them something like, "Listen, I know I always cancel, but I really want to make this happen this weekend. If I try to flake and cancel, don't let me get away with it!" I know at least some of my friends who would really like the opportunity to boss me around, so maybe I should give it to them.

Therapist: It sounds like your friends really care about you – that's great. If you think that will work for you in the short run, it seems like it's worth a try. What do you think?

Patient: Yes, I think so.

Therapist: What if you were to text them about it right now?

Patient: Right now???

Therapist: Well I'm hearing that you think it will help you follow through if you loop them in sooner rather than later. No time like the present.

Patient: OK, you're right. I'll do that now...

This strategy of brainstorming cognitive and behavioral barriers to following through on behavioral activation items can help to set the patient up for success.

Tips for the First Behavioral Activation Practice

People struggling with depression can have a difficult time reaping the rewards of behavioral activation exercises. Common difficulties are described in Table 7.

Table 7. Difficulties with behavioral activation for patients with PTSD and comorbid depression symptoms

Difficulty	Common pattern	Common solutions
Staying with the present moment	Getting distracted, worrying about the future, and thinking about the past.	Coach the participants to gently, nonjudgmentally redirect their attention back to the present moment repeatedly.
Discounting the positive	Patient reports "I enjoyed it some, but it used to be so much more fun."	Remind the patient to attempt to drop comparisons to the past. Highlight how the tendency to focus on cognitions about how things *should* feel prevents them from having permission to enjoy what is in front of them.
Savoring pleasant events	Patient reports having a hard time experiencing enjoyment during an activity.	Coach the patient to slow down and name what they are feeling in the moment.
Regret about the past	When the patient realizes that they are enjoying something, they start thinking "Why has it taken me so long to do this?" and feel frustrated.	Coach the patient to focus on the positive changes that they are making to improve their life from this point forward. Highlight how the tendency to focus on cognitions about what they *should* have been doing prevents them from ever starting new, healthy behaviors.

Processing Behavioral Activation Homework

The patient might complete the behavioral activation assignment and discover that they did not enjoy the activity or experience a sense of accomplishment from it. Rather than a "failed" homework, this helpful experiment allows the patient to brainstorm how to change the practice for the future to make it more enjoyable/rewarding. For any activities that the patient completed and enjoyed, it can be helpful to discuss *what* they enjoyed and *why* they enjoyed it, and to use this to make a plan to build on this momentum for the future.

Selecting Future Behavioral Activation Practices

After the initial behavioral activation session, it can be helpful to encourage the patient to "choose their own adventure" with future behavioral activation homework exercises. That includes helping them to focus on activities that would feel pleasurable, build a sense of self-efficacy or accomplishment, or simply feel like an investment in their self-worth or self-care. The goal is to work toward a sustainable mix of pleasurable/self-efficacy-building activities in which the patient will consistently invest time and effort. By the end of treatment, it is ideal for the patient to have experimented with a wide variety of activities that they anticipate might be helpful for behavioral activation so that they can narrow this list to include activities that are reliably experienced as helpful. By checking in on behavioral activation each week, it is easier for the patient to build new habits to support them as they graduate from therapy and transition into maintenance of their treatment gains.

Mixing Behavioral Activation With Exposure Practice

PE therapy incorporates behavioral activation items when building the initial *in vivo* exposure hierarchy. During the hierarchy-building process, when patients identify an item that is better characterized as behavioral activation (versus an *in vivo* exposure practice), the therapist asks the patient to rate their anticipated difficulty of the practice on a scale from 0–100, where 100 is the most difficult activity imaginable and a 0 is the easiest activity ever. If difficulty ratings are not ideal for a given item, it is also sometimes helpful to include anticipated pleasure ratings. While the patient might include these behavioral activation items in a hierarchy, they might choose to complete the activities out of order.

Compared to the preponderance of evidence supporting exposure therapy practices for reducing PTSD symptoms, there is less evidence that behavioral activation by itself is effective at reducing PTSD symptoms. However, numerous studies demonstrate the benefit of behavioral activation for reducing symptoms of depression, and as discussed previously, improvement in depression tends to predict improvement in PTSD and vice versa (Brown et al., 2019) among patients with a principal diagnosis of PTSD. Given the robust support for *in vivo* exposure practices, it is important to ensure that attention to behavioral activation does not detract from exposure practice. To accomplish this goal, it can be helpful to assign a 2:1 ratio of *in vivo* exposures and behavioral activation. Each week, the therapist and the patient might collaboratively agree upon two *in vivo* exposure practices, one behavioral activation practice, and ongoing imaginal (or sometimes interoceptive) exposure practice.

Summary

Behavioral activation can directly target depression symptoms among patients with PTSD and support them as they intentionally practice activities to improve pleasure and self-efficacy. The basic premise of behavioral activation is to recognize the relationship between how patients spend their time and their sense of pleasure/accomplishment/overall mood; collaboratively brainstorm activities that the patient feels might promote their sense of mastery/accomplishment; schedule the completion of these activities; practice staying in the moment and savoring the benefit of the practices; and repeat the behavioral activation practices until they result in the development of a new habit.

9 Elicitation and Processing of Trauma-Related Cognitions

As was briefly mentioned in Chapter 1, trauma-related cognitions have long been conceptualized as central to the development and maintenance of PTSD. With the release of the DSM-5 (American Psychiatric Association, 2013), trauma-related cognitions were officially recognized as a core symptom of PTSD with the addition of cluster D (negative cognitions and mood). Prior research in my laboratory (Brown et al., 2019) revealed that trauma-related cognitions were strongly correlated with overall symptom severity among patients entering PTSD treatment, and improvement in trauma-related cognitions was strongly associated with overall PTSD symptom improvement. All evidence-based CBT approaches for treating PTSD address trauma-related cognitions to varying degrees. In cognitive processing therapy (CPT; Resick et al., 2016), cognitive modification is the core treatment goal. In approaches that emphasize exposure as the core treatment component, including prolonged exposure (PE) therapy, cognitive change is recognized as a core therapeutic goal, although the way that cognitive changes are attempted differs from the treatment approach in CPT. Regardless of which evidence-based practice the therapist is using, it can be helpful to recognize some common trauma-related cognitions to optimally address the cognitions in treatment.

Direct Versus Indirect Challenging of Trauma-Related Cognitions

CPT uses a direct approach to challenging trauma-related cognitions. This involves the formal elicitation of trauma-related cognitions in thought records, identification of types of cognitive distortions ("stuck points"), and analysis of trauma-related cognitions using cognitive restructuring techniques. The CPT treatment manual (Resick et al., 2016) provides a very thorough and helpful guide on this process, which will not be reiterated here.

Types of Trauma-Related Cognitions

The Posttraumatic Cognitions Inventory (PTCI) is a well-validated assessment of common trauma-related cognitions (Foa et al., 1999). The measure has three core subscales - namely, negative cognitions about the self, self-blame, and negative cognitions about the world. In this section, we will discuss common examples of these cognition subtypes and therapeutic approaches to address them in treatment.

Negative Thoughts About Oneself

Disempowerment

When an individual has a threatening experience in which they have little or no control over their environment, it is more likely that the experience will be coded as traumatic to the survivor (Foa et al., 1992). With exposure to repeated threatening experiences in which the survivor cannot control the outcome, learned helplessness can develop (Bargai et al., 2007; Hammack et al., 2012). According to Martin Seligman's famous research on this topic (Seligman, 1972), learned helplessness is defined by a pattern of cognitions and behaviors that emerge after repeated exposures to circumstances in which a person's behavior cannot prevent a bad outcome. Following such repeatedly defeating experiences, the subject perceives their behavior as ineffective, even when the rules of engagement change, such that the subject can exert control over their environment. In the experimental literature, this tendency to give up even when an animal might be able to escape from a bad outcome is described as "conservation-withdrawal" (Minor et al., 2011).

When a human being is exposed to a traumatic event where their power is stripped from them, it is common to start to believe that nothing they do can prevent bad things from happening to them. With this cognitive schema activated, people start to narrow their behavioral repertoire and limit their activities. They might abandon ambitions that they cherished prior to the trauma(s) because of a new perception that nothing that they do will ever matter. They might take up less space in social settings or default to blending in and submissive behaviors. They might take less precautionary measures toward their health because of a perspective that "bad things happen no matter what I do," which can backfire and result in missed opportunities for early prevention of medical comorbidities. (Indeed, patients with PTSD experience significantly higher rates of medical comorbidities, see Chapter 1). These choices make perfect sense for a person who views their behavior as meaningless and ineffectual. The self-fulfilling prophecy is often the heartbreaking consequence of a capable person viewing themselves as completely disempowered, because the more that a person believes they are not capable, the less that they do, and, in turn, the less capable they feel. Behavioral experiments, including exposure practice and behavioral activation, provide ideal opportunities to gather objective evidence to evaluate the veracity of disempowerment cognitions. As described in Chapter 5, the ideal behavioral experiment starts with elicitation of expectations (hypotheses) about the experiment before it commences. A patient with PTSD might have a hypothesis that if they encounter triggers about the trauma they will unravel and be completely unable to regulate themselves. Indeed, fears about unraveling cause the patient to avoid as many reminders of the trauma as possible, which causes the self-fulfilling prophecy effect, as the patient's behavioral repertoire shrinks with each avoidance choice. Exposure allows for a reversal of this cycle and promotes an opportunity for the patient to directly confront their feared triggers to evaluate whether their disempowering hypothesis about unraveling is reality-based. (Sometimes they also need support in defining what unraveling is, and how experiencing uncomfortable emotions is not synonymous with their feared mental breakdown.) After the exposure, the goal is to process the learning by following the patient's lead and supporting them in sharing their genuine reactions. In PE, the recommendation is to start processing following imaginal exposure with a reiteration of praise for doing the exercise, immediately followed by the same prompt each time: *What was that like for you?* Then, the therapist follows the patient's lead in discussing their reactions to the exposure practice. If the patient discusses their emotional reactions, the exposure itself, the memory of the trauma, or what they are feeling in the moment of processing, they are on the right track. The objective in this processing is to gather data about cognitions that come up repeatedly for the patient, which is one indication of a particularly important trauma-related cognition that is keeping the patient "stuck."

Once the therapist has identified that the patient has a core trauma-related cognition about disempowerment, the goal is to bring this cognition to light and to examine it by discussing it aloud with a curious and nonjudgmental approach. Some therapists might take the tack of asking the patient to conduct a formal cognitive-restructuring exercise with the cognition and to thoroughly evaluate the data in favor of the cognitions, followed by evaluating the data refuting the cognition before ultimately deciding on the accuracy of the thought. Other therapists might prefer the approach of inquiries about the utility of the thought – that is, whether the thought is helping the patient to get closer to their goals. In either approach, cognitive restructuring can follow. In cognitive restructuring, the goal could be to generate a thought that is more balanced/accurate or a thought that is more helpful for achieving the patient's goals. The cognitive therapist might follow this exercise with the generation of a coping card to write down the more accurate or more helpful thought (electronically or as a hard copy) so that the patient can access this thought more easily the next time that the original, disempowering cognition is generated.

In PE therapy, the approach to address trauma-related cognitions is less direct than using formal analysis of the accuracy or utility of the thought. Following an exposure therapy practice, the therapist works to elicit relevant cognitions that are keeping the patient stuck with their PTSD. The therapist will ask questions about the meaning of the trauma, including stimulus elements and responses during the trauma itself, as well as about the meaning of reactions that are happening to the trauma currently. As it relates to perceptions about disempowerment, the therapist will be on the lookout for core cognitions in this domain (e.g., "Nothing I do matters"; "I'm weak"; "What is the point of trying?"). When the therapist hears the patient repeating these types of cognitions frequently, they might reflect that back to the patient. For instance, the therapist might say: *I've noticed that you have mentioned how weak you are a few times since I've known you.* Alternatively, the therapist might follow up with an invitation to elaborate (*Tell me more about why you see yourself as such a weak person*) or even a targeted question to elicit a connection between the trauma and the cognitions (*Where* do *you think you learned that?* or *How did what you went through influence your thinking on that?*).

In PE therapy, patients audio-record their therapy sessions and listen to them between sessions. Specifically, they listen to their imaginal exposure daily and the full session, including processing, at least once. As they listen intently to themselves talk about the most painful events that ever happened to them, cognitive shifts start to occur. Patients often report that as they hear themselves talk about what they went through, they start to have a lot more empathy for themselves (there will be more on this topic in the next section, on thoughts about being defective). They also report that they start to make new connections about their lives, such as how when they hear themselves talk, they can hear themes about disempowerment that are predetermining their choices.

A patient might notice, "When I talk about myself as totally weak, it's almost like I've accepted defeat. I want more for myself, so I have to figure out a way out of this mindset." This revelation allows the therapist to follow up with open-ended questions about what they want to do to change this mindset. For instance, the therapist might ask, *How are you going to figure this out?* or *What would you need to do to convince you that you aren't defeated?*

Another patient might report: "I hear myself talk about how nothing matters, and it doesn't matter what I do. But then I realize that if that were true,

I probably wouldn't be trying to make my life better. It's a bit hypocritical." The therapist might respond to this with a reflection such as, *It seems like you are stuck between deciding that nothing matters and deciding that you want to build a different future for yourself.* Alternatively, the therapist might follow this line of thinking by asking, *What do you want your life to be about? How are you going to get there?*

Sometimes the therapist might need to increase the intensity of communication about disempowering cognitions to support the patient in regaining their empowerment. For instance, after reflecting the disempowerment cognitions to the patient, the therapist might need to help the patient dig deeper by asking, *It seems like you have decided that you are completely weak and because you have decided that, it makes you want to give up. It's really hard to keep going when you see yourself that way. How are you going to break free from this type of thinking?*

Patients with PTSD very commonly struggle with disempowering cognitions about themselves that can unnecessarily keep them stuck in suffering. In addition to doing the cognitive refutation strategies described above, which are both direct and indirect, patients can also abandon this style of thinking by taking chances to build their confidence through behavioral experiments such as *in vivo* exposure and behavioral activation. Patients thrive when their therapy allows for ample opportunities to build their independence and self-confidence.

Shame/Feeling Defective

Patients with PTSD often struggle with significant shame, which results in cognitions about being a bad person, being defective, or having something deeply wrong with them. These cognitions can take the form of being irreparably damaged because of the trauma. In some cases of sexual trauma, the irreparable damage takes the form of also being unclean, contaminated, or "gross." When the patient sustains an injury or scar because of their trauma, these injuries might further reinforce their beliefs about being defective.

In some cases of childhood sexual trauma, the survivor of the trauma might have complicated emotional reactions to the physical sensations that they experienced during the trauma. When a child is sexually abused, the physical sensations that accompany the abuse can run the full spectrum from physical pain to physical pleasure. When a person experiences pleasure during sexual abuse but later develops PTSD from the abuse, they might have an extremely complicated cognitive reaction to this dichotomy that takes the form of feeling defective. For instance, a patient may believe, "There must be something wrong with me because there were parts of the experience that I enjoyed." In some situations, a child might not perceive that sexual abuse is traumatic at the time of its occurrence and might struggle with how to reconcile this with their current understanding of what is socially acceptable.

In addition, survivors of childhood sexual abuse might be drawn to or repelled by the perpetrator of the abuse. When survivors are drawn to the perpetrator prior to the abuse, they initially might feel special, that they were "chosen" by the perpetrator during the abuse. In some instances, perpetrators reinforce this message by telling children these messages directly (e.g., "I want to do these secret things with you because you're special"). Most children desire special attention from adults, yet the survivor of childhood sexual abuse might think that they are defective for craving such attention. Perpetrators of abuse often prey on children by capitalizing on their desire for more adult attention. In turn, adult survivors of childhood sexual abuse end up thinking that there is something wrong with them for having been drawn to the perpetrator of abuse.

The shame driving these cognitions often encourages patients with PTSD to hide for fear that others will discover their failings. Because of the desire for self-preservation, patients with PTSD often keep their perceived failings to themselves, providing little opportunity for them to get new data about the inaccuracy of their perceptions. Accordingly, their perceptions about being defective go unchecked and shame continues to increase over time.

Given the pattern of having shameful cognitions and then feeling the need to keep them private, the goal for PTSD-focused therapies is to support the patient is disclosing their perceived failings, shedding light on them, and discussing them openly to reduce their impact on the patient. The same approaches as for addressing disempowering cognitions apply to defective cognitions; therapists could opt to engage in traditional cognitive restructuring to evaluate the accuracy/helpfulness of the thoughts, or they could simply encourage the patient to discuss the thoughts out loud and listen to themselves talk about them on the audio recording to change their relationship to the thoughts.

Given the shameful cycle of thoughts about being defective, some patients do not feel comfortable disclosing their thoughts until they have got to know and trust the therapist over several sessions. This is one of the reasons why it is essential to assume that our initial conceptual model for a patient's suffering is potentially inaccurate and open to refinement as we gather more data. In PE, it can be helpful to enter into the processing of an exposure without an agenda to allow for these cognitions to emerge if the patient feels comfortable. It is not uncommon to go through two or three processing discussions (following an imaginal exposure) with a patient and for the therapist to remain confused about what exactly is keeping the patient stuck with their trauma in terms of negative cognitions. It is common that when therapists feel confused about what is keeping the patient stuck, a core cognition about being defective is part of the patient's core trauma-related cognitive schema. In cases where a therapist suspects a defective cognition plays a part, it can sometimes be helpful to openly explore this possibility using normalizing, for instance: *A lot of patients with whom I have worked have really complicated thoughts about themselves after the trauma. Some think that the trauma ruined them forever, or that it happened because there is something wrong with them. Others are embarrassed about something that they did or felt during the trauma. Do any of those things resonate with you?*

Other patients are so entrenched in their beliefs about being defective that they rehearse these cognitions out loud with the therapist beginning in the initial intake assessment and continuing thereafter. For these patients, it can be helpful to catch ruminative thinking patterns in their tracks and to help the patient to break free from negative thinking spirals. For instance, the therapist might remark, *I notice that you are often* very *critical of yourself in our sessions together. Do I have your permission to point out to you when I notice that you are falling into that spiral so that I can help you get unstuck?*

Self-Blame

Patients with PTSD very commonly blame themselves for the trauma or for what happened in its aftermath. The core cognitions that tend to emerge in this domain fall under the categories of responsibility and perceptions about what the patient deserves in the future.

Responsibility

Cognitions about blameworthiness are a core symptom of PTSD, separate from general changes in trauma-related cognitions. Patients with PTSD sometimes perceive that they did something to cause the trauma in the first place. For example, a patient might believe that they should not have been where they were when the trauma happened, or that they should not have worn what they were wearing, been with who they were with, or said or done something that they think contributed to the trauma. They also might believe that they should have told someone about a trauma sooner so that someone could have helped them, even in instances where they were threatened about the implications of disclosing what happened to them. Sometimes patients get messages from the outside context that further reinforces their self-blame, including when they hear how other trauma survivors are discussed in the media or in their community. When survivors of trauma hear other people engaging in victim (survivor) blaming about another person or raising criticisms of other survivors for not reporting their stories earlier, these communications can become internalized by the survivors themselves, who view a similarity between their own stories and a person who is being unfairly blamed for their trauma or its aftermath.

Sometimes survivors of trauma relate to cognitions about how the person feels that they should have said "no" more forcefully to a person perpetrating a trauma toward them. Because trauma memories are imperfect and often fragmented, survivors of trauma will sometimes forget how much effort they exerted to fight back against an assailant. This is one of the reasons why it can be helpful to support the patient in retelling the story of their trauma through imaginal exposure, which allows the patient to think through the context of what happened to them, what was said and done to them, and how they reacted. Also, in some cases, a survivor of trauma might not have fought against a perpetrator because fighting back would have been more dangerous for themselves or someone else. Despite the appropriateness of a decision to engage in submissive behavior for the sake of survival during the trauma, the survivor might continue to blame themselves for this behavior or feel tremendous shame about it.

Another common self-blaming theme that comes up for survivors of trauma emerge when a survivor of trauma knows of other people who were harmed in a similar manner. Sometimes patients believe that they should have done more to stop a perpetrator of trauma toward themselves in order to have prevented the perpetrator from engaging in the same behavior toward other people. This can sometimes come up in the context of childhood sexual abuse when a perpetrator for a patient also abused another family member (e.g., a sibling, cousin) or close friend. The patient may believe that they should have been more proactive about stopping the perpetrator. This belief system can dominate the patient's thinking even when there were obvious barriers to stopping the perpetrator. For instance, even when the perpetrator threatened the patient, the patient may still believe that they should have taken a more active stance against the perpetrator.

When these self-blame cognitions emerge, it can be helpful to support the patient in remembering what it was like for them to be in their own shoes when the trauma occurred. Trying to really visualize what it was like to be the age that they were and in the circumstances that they were in during the trauma can help the person to reduce their self-blame. When the trauma occurred during childhood or adolescence, it can be helpful for the patient to do an exposure wherein they associate with people who are the same age as the patient during the trauma. For instance, when working with a patient who was abused at the age of 7, it might help to ask, *When was the last time that you were around a 7-year-old? What are they like? What does that mean about what you were like at 7?* Occasionally, patients will push back on this line of questioning by saying, "I should have known better even if other 7-year-olds do not." Sometimes it can be helpful to inquire about whether they would apply the same level of responsibility that they apply to themselves to children they know. For instance, *If your nephew was abused like this, would you assume that he was to blame?* In such cases, it might be helpful to further unearth the cognitions that drive this belief and that cause the patient to hold themselves to a higher standard than other people. Once those cognitions are discussed out loud, the logic underlying them usually starts to crumble and the cognition becomes less sticky.

Deserving Bad Outcomes

For some survivors of trauma, themes of responsibility are so significant that they start to believe that they deserve negative outcomes in the future. For instance, some survivors will report that they do not deserve happiness after the trauma. This is especially prominent when the patient has survivor's guilt following a trauma in which other parties were significantly harmed or even died. Some survivors will resort to engaging in a style of punishing themselves for what they believe to be mistakes that they made (intentionally or not) that resulted in harm to others. The form of punishment that a particular patient takes can manifest itself as self-harm behaviors, limiting engagement in activities that might be enjoyable, limiting career progression or intimacy with a potential romantic partner, and other adverse outcomes.

Some patients might not recognize that they are punishing themselves but might notice that they feel guilty when they enjoy positive life experiences or feel overwhelmed with sadness after positive events because of a realization that their loved one is missing out on the experience. By encouraging the patient to discuss these cognitions out loud, the logic in the cognition might start to unravel, allowing for more adaptive interpretations. For instance, the patient might hear themselves saying these extreme cognitions and later react with: "As I hear myself saying these things, it makes me really sad. It also makes me realize that this is so not what [my deceased husband] would want for me. It's hard to shake the thought that I don't deserve happiness without him, but I know that I need to try."

Other patients might require more effortful processing of these deep-rooted beliefs for them to build insight into their problematic nature. Some intervention opportunities to support emotional processing of these difficult scenarios are described in Table 8.

Table 8. Support with cognitively processing guilt-based cognitions

Type of intervention	Intervention suggestion
Reflection	Reflect back to the patient what you hear, for instance, "I'm hearing that you feel you need to stay stuck in the past in order for things to be fair or just. Is that what you mean?"
Metaphor	PE (Foa et al., 2007, 2019) makes reference to a "guilt jail" for individuals who are struggling with guilt following a trauma. For instance: "You have been stuck in a state of misery about this scenario for so long – it's almost like you are keeping yourself locked in a guilt jail to make up for what's happened. Does that sound right to you? I'm wondering when you think it's appropriate to let yourself out of that jail?"
Focus on a constructive, meaningful plan	Patients sometimes get stuck in a negative thought spiral about guilt and one way to support them in getting out of it is asking them what they need to get unstuck. For instance: "What would need to happen for you to give yourself permission to move forward in your life? What concrete steps could we take to help get you there?"
Comparisons to other people	Advise patients to compare the standard that they apply to themselves to the standards that they apply to others. Sometimes it can be helpful to ask whether the patient would have the same expectations of another person that they hold for themselves. It is most helpful to select a comparison person whom the patient loves. For instance: "If your daughter were driving in her car with a friend, someone else ran a red light, and her friend passed away, would you think that your daughter deserved to keep herself in a state of guilt jail for years to come? Why not? Why is it the case that you hold yourself to another standard than you hold her?" When this line of questioning is insufficient, it can sometimes be helpful to assign homework to further the learning. For instance, you might assign the patient to list 10 reasons why they should be held to a higher standard than their daughter, or 10 reasons why other people deserve forgiveness but they themselves do not.

These interventions include reflecting the core theme of lack of self-forgiveness back to the patient, using metaphor to illustrate the dilemma, focusing on a concrete path for the patient to move forward, and using comparisons to others to highlight unrealistic standards for themselves.

Negative Thoughts About the World

In addition to general negative thoughts about themselves and self-blame, survivors of PTSD commonly struggle with negative thoughts about the world. These thoughts can pervade relationships with intimate partners, work colleagues, friends, roommates, and neighbors. I bucket these types of thoughts into two global categories: cognitions about trust and about burdensomeness.

Inability to Trust Others

Following a trauma, particularly a trauma that involved perpetration of harm by another person, it is common for survivors with PTSD to report having less trust in other people. While this is an understandable cognitive reaction to experiencing psychological and/or physical harm, it can prevent a deepening of relationships with others and result in significant impairment for survivors. The ability to trust people, within reason, is foundational to relationship building. In the absence of a capacity to trust others, interactions become surface level and unfulfilling for both parties. A superficial relationship sometimes results in other people interpreting the trauma survivor as uninterested in connection and leads them to slowly back out of the survivor's life. This fizzling of a relationship ultimately confirms the trauma survivor's perception that other people cannot be trusted, resulting in a greater need to pull back from intimate connections.

To build an intimate connection requires some level of vulnerable expression by both parties. When a trauma survivor has a history of being abused or taken advantage of, it is unsurprising that they might feel extremely uncomfortable with showing vulnerability. In fact, some survivors of trauma might believe that something about their younger selves was interpreted as vulnerable by a perpetrator of trauma, further reinforcing the need to come across as strong and guarded. An inability to trust anyone results in reinforcement of shame and worsening of negative cognitions about the self. Specifically, when a trauma survivor experiences embarrassment, they might be more reluctant to disclose that embarrassment to other people. Hiding embarrassing details prevents opportunities for others to validate an experience by normalizing or providing support. The more a person hides, the more they feel convinced that they have something to hide, further reinforcing the shame.

The recommendation for trust building is to encourage the trauma survivor to select one or two seemingly trustworthy people and to practice gradually opening up to them with low-stakes personal disclosures. Sometimes these vulnerability exercises are officially included on an *in vivo* exposure hierarchy, and they can start with seemingly trivial exercises. To begin, patients may practice expressing a genuine opinion rather than "going with the flow" of others. Based on the results of this behavioral experiment, the survivor might decide to gradually disclose a bit more about their genuine feelings about things. Over time, as more trust is built, they might choose to disclose more personal details about their life. The decision about what to share and who to share it with should always remain with the patient so that they feel empowered to remain in control of their story.

Some survivors of trauma have an altered threat detector following the trauma so that they might become *too trusting* of individuals who have not earned their trust. This can sometimes occur when a child is exposed to repeated instances of abuse or neglect and learns that their environment is very unsafe, and it might help their survival if they latch onto *anyone,* given that it is impossible for them to trust people whom they should be able to trust. Other survivors of trauma have witnessed family members suffer abuse in intimate partner violence and have come to interpret such violence as an expected part of being in a family. Survivors of families with intimate partner violence might trust new partners who display a propensity to abuse because they have learned that violence is a predictable part of being close to others. Given that trauma exposure can change propensity to threat in either direction, it can be important to coach patients to evaluate the safety of vulnerable disclosure to or closeness with partners through an ongoing analysis of the data supporting versus refuting the trustworthiness of a particular partner. When a patient is actively involved in a relationship characterized by intimate partner violence, the therapist and patient must carefully assess the appropriateness of engaging in PTSD therapy. For more details, see Chapter 11.

Perceptions of Being a Burden to Others

PTSD can convince survivors of trauma that other people would be better off without them and that they are a burden on their loved ones. Sometimes the beliefs of burdensomeness are reinforced in individuals who need to take leaves of absence from work or who, in the case of active-duty service members, might need to leave their jobs altogether due to the lasting repercussions of trauma exposure. Burdensomeness is independently associated with suicide risk (Joiner, 2005) and can contribute to attempts to isolate from other people, creating more loneliness and despair.

Some trauma survivors come to believe that the trauma ruined them and their ability to regulate their reactions, including anger-driven reactions. Individuals with PTSD are often worried about lashing out in anger at other people, whether or not they have engaged in violent behaviors in the past. When an individual with PTSD expresses anger or irritability, they might become overwhelmed with regret and use this reaction as evidence that they bring harm to those whom they love. When a patient with PTSD is very worried about expressions of irritability, they might go to great lengths to avoid their family, especially when they are upset. This can cause them to miss out on important events, causing the family to express discontent and further increasing anger in the trauma survivor. Many, but not all, people with PTSD are *irrationally* obsessed with fears about what they might do when they become angry. This is particularly true in survivors of combat trauma or individuals who have a history of violence exposure. In these cases, it is essential to assess whether the patient has engaged in violent acts outside the context of the trauma and, if so, under what circumstances. If the patient has a history of perpetrating intimate partner violence, it might be optimal to consider a therapy focused on anger management before proceeding with PTSD-focused therapy. For more details on this topic, refer to Chapter 11. Alternatively, if a patient has no history of violence against family or close friends, they might need to practice exposure to difficult emotions, even in the context of loved ones, to have a corrective learning opportunity ("I can feel negative emotions and not lash out in anger").

Disconnection/Perceptions of Being an Outsider

A core symptom of PTSD is a feeling of disconnection from other people. Some patients with PTSD describe this as though there is a wall between them and other people. The sense of disconnection from others can stem from a perception that other people cannot possibly understand what it is like to have gone through what the patient went through, a perception that might be based in reality. Feeling like an outsider to others can also come from negative perceptions about oneself or shame about being inadequate or unworthy of love from or closeness to others. Perceptions of being in the "outgroup" can be reinforced when disclosures about the trauma to other people are brushed off, not believed, or assumed to be an exaggeration of reality. These experiences further convince a patient with PTSD that they should keep to themselves, that other people cannot be trusted, and that other people are not like them.

Perceptions of being an outsider are common among survivors of PTSD who have left the context in which the original trauma occurred. For example, refugees who flee their home countries to escape from violence have multiple odds stacked against them in terms of building a new network or "in group" in their new home. These can include the PTSD symptoms that bring them to treatment, the fact that they are in a new culture with customs that they are not comfortable with, and in many cases, the need to learn a new language, which can promote more feelings of alienation. Another example is a survivor of combat trauma who feels like an outsider to their home community upon return from deployment. Whereas they might have experienced unit cohesion while deployed, the sense of closeness is lost when they return from deployment, and the survivor with PTSD faces an uphill battle. Not only are they struggling with the PTSD symptoms that bring them to the therapist's office for treatment, but they might be living in a community that does not understand the military culture, PTSD symptoms, or the effects of deployment and trauma exposure.

For anyone struggling with a sense of feeling like part of the "out group" as part of their PTSD experience, it can be essential to slowly build closeness or reconnect with their community. It might be necessary for patients to redefine their community and select trustworthy people with whom they want to develop closeness. Community-building efforts can be incorporated as part of *in vivo* exposure exercises or behavioral activation as relevant.

Summary

PTSD develops in part due to negative trauma-related cognitions about the self, other people, and the world. These cognitions become further reinforced when patients with PTSD are overwhelmed by their negative emotions and do not push themselves to conduct behavioral experiments to push the limits of their belief system. By becoming more aware of these cognitions and consciously practicing gathering data about their veracity, either through formal cognitive exercises or behavioral experiments, trauma-related cognitions can become more flexible and adaptive over time.

10 Managing Suicide Risk in the Treatment of PTSD

PTSD significantly increases risk for suicidal ideation (Brown, Fernandez, et al., 2018; Kratovic et al., 2021; Tarrier & Gregg, 2004), suicide attempts (Stevens et al., 2013; Tarrier & Gregg, 2004), and death by suicide (Gradus et al., 2010; Krysinska & Lester, 2010). The mechanisms underlying the association between PTSD and suicide risk can include increased depression severity, negative cognitions about other people (a critical feature of many theories about the development of suicidal ideation; Joiner, 2005; Klonsky & May, 2015), changes in arousal (Brown, Contractor, et al., 2018; Brown et al., 2020), changes in cognitive control (Bredemeier & Miller, 2015; Herzog et al., 2019), and even changes in factors that increase possession of lethal means, such as firearms, though the research on this topic is very mixed (Betz et al., 2023). Given the strong association between PTSD and suicide risk, it is essential to consider how best to mitigate suicide risk before, during, and after PTSD treatment.

Understanding Suicide Risk in the Context of PTSD

People, including those with PTSD, can experience rapid changes in suicidal ideation and urges to engage in suicide attempts over even short windows of time (Brown, Zhu, et al., 2022; Zhu et al., 2022). Many suicidologists argue against the concept of differentiating participants into categories of risk (Bryan et al., 2020). This is because rather than risk constituting a static and reliable characteristic, it fluctuates significantly within and between patients over time, as is reflected in the fluid vulnerability theory of suicide (Rudd, 2006).

Clinicians might feel more comfortable if they can confidently categorize a particular patient into a "high-risk" or "low-risk group." Such classifications might provide reassurance to a clinician that a particular low-risk patient is unlikely to make a suicide attempt between sessions, thereby reducing the need for being available for responding to crises. If a therapist is out of practice with appropriately responding to suicide risk (or never learned how to), they might experience increased fear and discomfort with this topic. The therapist might inadvertently communicate their discomfort to the patient with conversations about suicide. For example, a therapist who is uncomfortable with assessing suicide risk might ask their patient, *You haven't been thinking about suicide, have you?* Alternatively, a clinician might couch assessments of suicide risk with offputting warnings before the question (*Now I'm going to ask you some questions that I ask everyone, even if I don't think it's relevant to you*), which guides the patient to deny suicidal ideation. More discussion about strategies for appropriately assessing suicide risk among patients with PTSD is included later in this chapter.

When a therapist decides that their patient is low risk, this opens up the patient and the therapist to other problematic patterns of behavior. Some therapists only assess suicide risk during their initial assessment, whereas it is more appropriately assessed in an ongoing manner. Other therapists might decide to not inquire about access to lethal means in the absence of suicide risk, which limits opportunities to collaboratively discuss safe storage practices. Patients might be reluctant to discuss their firearms, even if they have concerns about safety, when a therapist does not initiate a conversation about the topic. Furthermore, if the therapist conveys a judgmental attitude toward the patient for their possession of a firearm, this will likely damage rapport and reduce the effectiveness of treatment (if the patient is even willing to continue treatment). More considerations for lethal means safety are discussed later in this chapter. Finally, when a therapist decides that their patient is low risk, they might start to adopt a laissez-faire attitude toward safety considerations, such as knowing the address where the patient is having their telehealth session. To assume that suicide risk is off the table for a patient sets up the therapeutic relationship and efficacy for failure.

In contrast, when a clinician encounters a patient that they categorize as "high risk," they might be more likely to simply refuse to provide treatment for the patient and to refer them elsewhere, even if the patient does not have optimal alternative referrals. In clinical practice, patients who are deemed "high risk" will frequently be referred to begin dialectical behavior therapy (DBT; Linehan, 1993) and demonstrate that their risk is stabilized before beginning treatment for PTSD. DBT is associated with reduced risk of suicide attempts in higher-risk samples (Linehan et al., 2015; McCauley et al., 2018). However, DBT is an intensive, expensive, and lengthy treatment that was developed for borderline personality disorder. Most individuals who struggle with suicidal ideation do not meet criteria for borderline personality disorder, just as many individuals who die by suicide do not have any known psychiatric illness (Stone, 2018). Therefore, it might be inappropriate to refer a patient for DBT based on suicidal ideation alone (in the absence of other symptoms of borderline personality disorder). In fact, two recent studies demonstrated that components of DBT could be iatrogenic in samples for which the treatment was not originally designed (e.g., in universal prevention approaches in schools; Harvey et al., 2023). Thus, referring some patients with suicide risk to DBT is not an ideal outcome.

In addition, when a patient presents for treatment for PTSD but is recommended to receive an alternative treatment prior to starting PTSD treatment, it might dissuade them from continuing in care at all. Some patients have a small window of willingness to initiate treatment, and if it takes too long to begin an appropriate treatment this can actually worsen their outcomes (Clark et al., 2009; Punton et al., 2022). Furthermore, if suicidal ideation is the result of symptoms of underlying PTSD-related distress, a much more efficient treatment plan would target the PTSD symptoms as soon as possible. If a therapist decides that they cannot start PTSD treatment with a patient until the patient's suicide risk is resolved, treatment might never commence.

Assessing Suicide Risk

Be Aware of the Consequences of a Patient Reporting Imminent Suicide Risk

It is common (and even adaptive) for patients to fear the consequences of honest disclosure of suicide risk. Even in my research studies that advertise to recruit participants based on suicidal ideation, participants are often nervous to be completely forthcoming about suicidal thinking and behaviors. Some participants and patients have disclosed traumatic consequences of honest disclosures about suicide risk. For instance, one participant shared the following (paraphrased for anonymity): "I told a mental health provider about my suicidal thoughts before, and they locked me up. It felt like a trap – they asked me about it, I was honest (including that I was *not* going to act on those thoughts), and the next thing I know, I'm being carted to the hospital by the police."

In many healthcare systems that have a security team, there are protocols for transportation of patients for involuntary commitment. Sometimes those protocols mandate handcuffing the patients (purportedly for their own safety and the safety of the security team). Even in the absence of being handcuffed, when transport to the hospital occurs in the back of a police car, patients commonly feel that their honest disclosure about suicide risk is being criminalized. Even for people who have not directly experienced these consequences, they may have people in their social network who were seemingly "punished" for honest disclosures about suicide risk, even by well-meaning healthcare systems and clinicians.

If you are doing clinical work with patients who have PTSD, it is essential to be aware of the full spectrum of possible consequences for your patients who disclose suicidal ideation. For those patients who require more thorough evaluation by a psychiatric emergency team, it is extremely helpful if you know about that process. Table 9 includes a checklist of items to help you familiarize yourself with the emergency psychiatric response options where you live.

Table 9. Things to know about your local emergency psychiatric response options

Issue	Key point(s)	Things to investigate
Availability of beds	Not all hospitals have inpatient psychiatric beds; in cities with different inpatient psychiatric facilities, your patient will likely be transported to a facility based on the availability of a bed for them.	Which facilities that have inpatient psychiatric beds are closest to your practice?
Psychiatric crisis response centers versus emergency departments	While a person can present to any emergency department with a psychiatric crisis, they might be transferred to a psychiatric crisis response center before they are thoroughly evaluated. For psychiatric evaluations that the emergency department deems are not urgent, they might encourage the patient to transport themselves to the psychiatric crisis response center.	Are there psychiatric crisis response centers where you live, and if there is more than one, which is closest to where your patient lives? Explain to your patient that they are welcome to go to any emergency department, but that their experience will be more efficient if they go to one with the capacity to conduct a psychiatric evaluation for inpatient hospitalization.
Transport for an emergency psychiatric evaluation	Some locations have mobile crisis response teams that can provide support with transport to the hospital. As described previously, if a patient presents to a general emergency department, they might first be transferred to a psychiatric crisis response center. If deemed appropriate for psychiatric inpatient admission, they may then be transferred again to a facility with an open bed.	Does your city have a mobile crisis team? If so, what services are available through the team? Who staffs the crisis team (e.g., clinicians, mental health support staff, police)? What services do they provide?

continued on next page

Table 9. Continued

Issue	Key point(s)	Things to investigate
Decisions about admission for a psychiatric hospitalization	For many psychiatric emergency evaluations, a positive outcome is one in which the patient is determined to be "safe" to be referred to outpatient care rather than admitted for a psychiatric hospitalization. When a patient presents to the emergency department/crisis response center for the first time, they might fully expect that the outcome of the evaluation will be hospitalization. They might even have psychologically prepared themselves for the hospitalization and feel invalidated if they are turned away.	Know what criteria are used to determine psychiatric hospitalization admission. Busy emergency clinicians (who often have more patients than beds available) will be most interested in assessing whether the patient is "safe" to return home. They may employ a strategy of retaining the patient in the crisis response center for some time (given that waiting is the norm rather than the exception anyway, as discussed next) to check in repeatedly about safety to determine whether the patient has returned to safety from a short-lived crisis. This is why it is essential not to recommend that a patient present for psychiatric emergency evaluation unless it is indicated. For example, is the patient expressing: suicidal ideation with a plan, intent, and a desire to imminently act on their plan? Those are typically the grounds for hospitalization. Anything less intense than these criteria will likely result in a referral back to outpatient care in many busy emergency centers.
Wait times	Depending on staff availability for assessment and bed availability, wait times can be longer than everyone prefers. This can be dysregulating for patients who might be having one of the worst days of their lives, prompting suicidal thoughts and behaviors.	It might be helpful to update patient expectations so that they are not surprised about a long wait.

continued on next page

Table 9. Continued

Issue	Key point(s)	Things to investigate
Waiting areas	Space is often at a premium in psychiatric emergency rooms. This may mean that the waiting areas are full and can be uncomfortable.	If the emergency area allows a family member to join the patient (not all do), it can be helpful to have someone with them for support. It can also be helpful to consider bringing along a book, a magazine, or something else for distraction. (Note that not all emergency areas allow patients to retain access to their phones.)

Building Rapport

A thorough suicide risk assessment is contingent upon establishing rapport. One way to start to build trust is to practice transparency with the patient about the goals for the suicide risk assessment.

Evidence-Based Assessment Strategies

Columbia-Suicide Severity Rating Scale (C-SSRS)

The C-SSRS (Posner et al., 2011) is a widely used assessment of the presence/absence of suicidal ideation, intensity of suicidal ideation, suicidal behavior, suicide attempts, and lethality of suicide attempts. During an initial evaluation of patients with PTSD, I recommend conducting a lifetime and past-month assessment of each of the three C-SSRS subscales. For patients with a significant history of suicidal ideation and behavior, it can be most efficient to use a self-report screener version of the C-SSRS before each session. Once the patient is familiar with the questions assessed by the C-SSRS, it can be even more efficient to ask them, *Have there been any changes in suicidal thinking or behavior since the last session?*

Self-Injurious Thoughts and Behaviors Interview–Revised (SITBI-R)

The SITBI-R (Fox et al., 2020) is a valuable, detailed alternative to the C-SSRS that has strong psychometric properties. I commonly use this assessment during research studies, as it allows for an in-depth exploration of multiple domains of important types of thinking and behavior patterns. Clinically, the full version of the measure is often too lengthy to implement in practice.

However, one of the valuable item types on the SITBI that is not reflected on the C-SSRS is an assessment of how likely participants think it will be that they will make a suicide attempt (or have other types of behaviors and thoughts) in the future. This type of question can assist the clinician in determining how the patient's current thinking about suicide might differ from their plans for the future.

Patient Health Questionnaire-9 (PHQ-9)

Many electronic health records have implemented the PHQ-9 (Kroenke et al., 2003) as a strategy for screening for suicide risk. However, relying exclusively on the PHQ-9 for evaluating the presence of suicidal thoughts is problematic because the assessment combines thoughts of death with thoughts of suicide. In addition, the PHQ-9 is not a strong predictor of future suicide attempts (Na et al., 2018).

Beck Scale for Suicide Ideation (BSS)

The BSS (Beck & Steer, 1991) is a 21-item self-report assessment of suicidal ideation and behavior. However, the first five items of the measure serve as a screen because participants who deny suicidal ideation do not complete the remaining questions. For this reason, this self-report assessment can provide a much more thorough assessment of suicidal ideation and behaviors relative to a single-item assessment commonly used in depression assessments.

Suicide-Visual Analog Scale (S-VAS)

The S-VAS (Bryan, 2019) provides an assessment of "urges to kill myself" on a 0–100-point sliding scale, where 0 is not at all and 100 is extreme. The measure has strong psychometric properties and predicts future suicide attempts (Bryan, 2019). In collaboration with Dr. Craig Bryan, I have used this tool during intensive daily assessment studies (Brown, Taylor, et al., 2022; Brown, Zhu, et al., 2022). In clinical practice, I have also administered the S-VAS immediately before and after an imaginal exposure practice for patients who are receiving PE therapy (Foa et al., 2007, 2019).

Appropriateness of Treatment for PTSD

Clinical practice guidelines long suggested against enrolling participants in PTSD-focused therapies, such as PE therapy, when patients were at increased risk for suicide (van Minnen et al., 2012). However, clinical trials had various interpretations of the level of suicide risk that warranted patients' exclusion from PTSD therapy. One of the challenges of determining PE appropriateness on the basis of suicide risk is that there is significant within-person variability of suicidal urges on a given day (Brown, Zhu, et al., 2022). Thus, a patient who denies significant suicidal ideation in your office might experience intense suicidal ideation an hour later for various reasons. And another hour later, the suicidal ideation might lessen significantly. This is further support for the futility of attempting to categorize participants into "low-risk" and "high-risk" groups.

One of the only studies that explored the safety of PE with patients who were at acute risk for suicide integrated the treatment with DBT (Linehan, 1993). In the first study on this topic, patients received DBT first and were required to abstain from self-injurious behavior and suicide attempts for at least 8 weeks prior to transitioning into PE (Harned et al., 2012, 2014). In that protocol, if a patient engages in self-injurious behavior or makes a suicide attempt after beginning PE, PE is paused and the clinical team reverts to DBT until an additional 8 weeks have passed without self-harm or suicide attempts (Harned et al., 2014). The limited data that are available for this integrated protocol demonstrated that compared to DBT alone, patients who received DBT–PE had significantly lower rates of suicide attempts and self-harm behaviors, as well as significantly greater reductions in PTSD symptom severity (Harned et al., 2014). However, much more research is needed to evaluate the efficacy of this integration in larger samples.

Harned and colleagues' (2014) offered the only empirical recommendation available in the literature about how long a patient should abstain from self-harm behavior and suicide attempts prior to beginning PE, and how long PE should be paused if self-harm or a suicide attempt occurs in treatment (8 weeks, in both cases). More research is needed to evaluate whether shorter time frames are safe for patients. Given that suicide risk is exacerbated by PTSD symptoms, we need more guidance on how to help patients get access to PTSD treatments as early as is safe and tolerable following self-harm or a suicide attempt.

Clinician Anxiety About Working With Patients With Significant Suicidal Ideation

Working with patients who are experiencing significant suicidal ideation can be frightening, even for very seasoned clinicians. Some clinicians cope with anxiety about suicide risk via denial. These clinicians might prefer to avoid conversations about suicide risk for fear that they will not know how to help the patient, or even make the suicide risk worse. Decades of evidence highlight that assessing suicide risk does not increase the risk of suicide (Bender et al., 2019). Assessing suicide risk does not "plant the seed" for someone to start thinking about suicide when they were not already thinking about it (Dazzi et al., 2014). Research from my lab has demonstrated that frequent assessment of suicide risk can reduce suicide risk in some patients who in qualitative explorations reported that by answering questions about their level of risk, they felt a sense of accountability to do something to make themselves feel better (Ballentine et al., 2025). On the other hand, when a clinician avoids discussions about suicide risk, the patient might interpret this avoidance as an indication that the clinician is not comfortable discussing the topic, so the patient will therefore not disclose high risk. For these and other reasons, it is unethical for clinicians to avoid talking about suicide risk with their patients.

Conversely, some clinicians have unrealistic expectations about how much control they can exert over their patients. A clinician might adopt a "God complex," where they attempt to micromanage and control a patient to prevent them from dying by suicide. Other than when a patient is reporting suicidal ideation with a plan and intent to imminently act on this plan (warranting consideration for hospitalization), a clinician should resist the urge to control the patient's behavior. Instead, a worthy and effective goal is to strive to understand the patient's suffering and provide them with emotional support, validation, and practical problem-solving strategies. Our ethical, moral, and legal obligations as mental health providers is to engage in evidence-based assessments of suicide risk, provide evidence-based interventions to reduce risk, and thoroughly document our reliance on gold-standard approaches. Even when clinicians follow this guidance, some of their patients will die by suicide. We cannot delude ourselves into trying to control people and situations that are outside of our control. Failing to stay grounded in what is in your control as a clinician is a recipe for burnout and for clinicians to make arbitrary decisions in their clinical practice, such as, *I don't treat patients who are at high risk for suicide.* This would be a loss for the field, your patients, and your community.

Safety Planning Intervention and Crisis Response Planning

The Stanley-Brown Safety Planning Intervention (Stanley et al., 2018) and crisis response planning (Bryan et al., 2017) are each evidence-based interventions to reduce risk for future suicide attempts. These interventions share an approach toward anticipating future crises; the interventions are both rooted in the idea that people who have experienced suicidal crises in the past will experience future suicidal crises. We know that when a person is in an emotional crisis (including a suicidal crisis), their problem-solving capacity is reduced (Gibbs et al., 2009; Williams et al., 2005). The rationale for both the Stanley-Brown Safety Planning Intervention and crisis response planning is that it can be valuable to anticipate future crises now, so that when the crisis emerges, the patient already has a plan to navigate it as safely as possible. Both interventions also rely on a collaborative conversation between the clinician and the patient to ensure that the plan is personalized to the unique needs of the patient. For clinicians who desire to learn more about these interventions, there are trainings available through the intervention developers.

Lethal Means Safety

The lethality of suicidal behavior is dictated by a combination of a person's intent underlying the behavior and the selection of a particular method. Nearly 90% of people who make a suicide attempt with a firearm die (Elnour & Harrison, 2008); in contrast, only 1.5–3.3% of people who use drugs/poisoning and 1.1–3.7% of people who use cutting as their method for a suicide attempt die (Elnour & Harrison, 2008). Many people who have one suicide method in mind do *not* switch to an alternative method when access to their preferred method is thwarted (Almeida et al., 2023; Deisenhammer et al., 2016). For this reason, lethal means safety interventions that put obstacles between a person and a suicide method to delay their access or make it slightly harder to access can significantly reduce the risk of death (Yip et al., 2012).

The goal for lethal means safety is to support patients with anticipating whether there are any realistic obstacles that they want to put between themselves and access to their preferred suicide method. For firearms, patients might opt to store their weapon in a locked gun safe, to store their ammunition separately from their weapon, to implement a gun lock (which often comes with handguns at the time of purchase and is generally inexpensive even if purchased on its own), to store their weapon in a gun storage facility, or to store their weapon with a trusted person. For patients with a preferred method of overdosing on medications, they might opt to receive weekly rather than monthly prescriptions of medications, to store their medications in daily dispenser plastic containers to make it more annoying to access many at a time, to have a trusted person control access to their medications, or to lock away access to their medications between dosages. Some patients might opt to get rid of their preferred method altogether; other patients might prefer to change how they access their method. Still other patients might benefit from having a list of reasons for living or a symbolic reminder of these reasons displayed near their suicide method.

It is common for the first conversation about lethal means safety to serve as a jumping-off point. The value in these conversations lies in starting to curiously explore options to promote safety without an agenda to impose on the patient. I caution clinicians against trying to rush their patients into storing their lethal means in an alternative manner, as this pressure can back-fire and lead to both parties feeling more polarized in their opinions. This is particularly important when the patient has access to a firearm and perceives that the therapist is simply "trying to get me to get rid of my gun" or is even being "antigun." The more collaborative the conversation, the greater the chance of a safer outcome in the long run.

Coping With Suicide Loss

Many clinicians lose a patient to suicide at some point in their career; I lost my first patient to suicide when I was a third-year graduate student. When I lost my patient, it had a profound impact on me personally and professionally. For those of you who have already lost a patient to suicide, my heart goes out to you, and I hope that you have found a way to make peace with this tragedy so that you can continue providing care to other patients and being present with your loved ones. I processed my grief over this loss with the support of an amazing team of supervisors at the time, who provided emotional support, validation, and practical support in the form of gift cards for self-care (admittedly, my best self-care at the time was a Slurpee, and I will never forget that my supervisor, Dr. Nancy Argueta, remembered that and brought me a gift card for it, which I still have).

For each of us who have patients who are struggling with suicide risk, I think that it is essential to have access to a nonjudgmental community of clinicians who understand this emotional rollercoaster. This is one of the reasons why in DBT, a consultation team is required for adherence to the therapeutic model (Linehan, 1993). For the audience reading this book, a group drawn to providing care to patients with PTSD, it can be even more important to find a community to help you with ethically sharing the burden of your important work.

Summary

Patients with PTSD are at significantly higher risk for suicide compared to the general population. In this chapter, I discussed strategies to build rapport in the context of assessing and intervening to reduce suicide risk among your patients with PTSD. I also discussed evidence-based suicide risk assessment strategies, including clinical interviews and self-report assessments. Brief interventions to reduce suicide risk were reviewed, including the Stanley-Brown Safety Planning Intervention and crisis response planning, as were strategies to consider for lethal means safety. Finally, I discussed considerations for supporting clinicians who have lost a patient to suicide.

11 Working With Survivors of Intimate Partner Violence

Estimates of the prevalence of intimate partner violence vary drastically based on the culture. Some studies have found that global prevalence estimates for women vary from 15–71%, depending on the country under study, with 4–51% reporting intimate partner violence in the past year alone (Garcia-Moreno et al., 2006). Prevalence rates for men are generally lower (approximately 20%), although not enough research has been directed toward this topic to make a genuine comparison (Kolbe & Büttner, 2020). Exposure to intimate

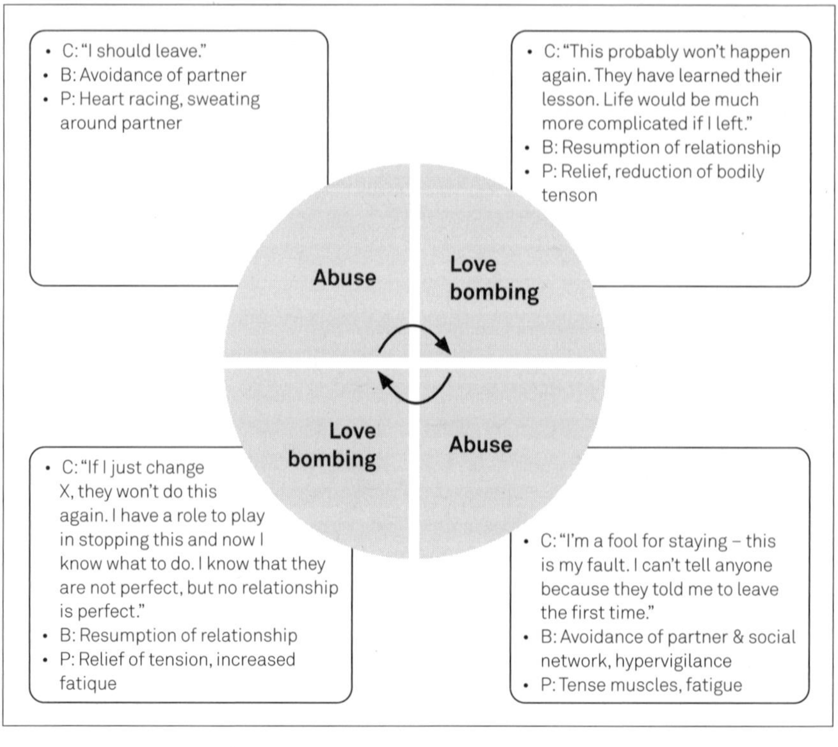

Figure 6. Cycle of abuse (C = common cognitions, B = common behaviors, P = common physical sensations).

partner violence can increase the likelihood of developing PTSD (White et al., 2024). Furthermore, up to 40% of survivors of intimate partner violence will go on to develop PTSD (Jones et al., 2001). Survivors of intimate partner violence commonly experience a recurring cycle of abuse, wherein a partner inflicts abuse and then attempts to repair the relationship with excessive displays of love and affection ("love bombing"), which convinces the survivor to stay in the relationship (Roddy & Dubrow-Marshall, 2023), before the next round of abuse is inflicted. An example of this cycle is depicted in Figure 6. This cycle of abuse results in repeated exposure to traumatic violent experiences.

Assessing Intimate Partner Violence

When your patient has come to therapy to work on distress related to violence in their relationship, it is essential to conduct a thorough assessment of the nature of the violence (Nicholls et al., 2013). In general, assessments of intimate partner violence do not outperform assessments of overall risk of violence in terms of predicting future exposure to violence (Nicholls et al., 2013). However, standardized assessments can confer clinical advantages for the patient. Some measures have been developed for deployment by police immediately following a case of violence, which are not as relevant here. Some evidence-based assessment measures that may be useful to incorporate in clinical practice include the Domestic Violence Evaluation (DOVE; Ellis & Stuckless, 2006), typically administered to couples, and the Danger Assessment Scale (Campbell et al., 2009). These standardized assessments can accomplish two goals: (1) performing a systematic screening of all clinic patients for the presence of violence; and (2) conveying to patients that you are comfortable discussing violence in their relationship and are therefore unlikely to either overreact to or minimize the experience. Thus, formal, standardized assessments of violence in the relationship are strongly recommended.

When a clinician chooses to assess for relationship violence informally, it is essential to do so with questions that do not imply a "correct" answer. For instance, a clinician might inappropriately ask, *There has never been violence in your relationship, right?* A patient immediately knows what the "right" answer to this question is, and they might pick up on how it would be easier for both the therapist and the patient if they denied the abuse. An alternative, more appropriate version of this assessment is, *Please tell me about times when you might have felt unsafe in your relationship* (open ended) or *Have there been times in your relationship when you have felt unsafe?* (closed ended). The risk of informal assessments is that the clinician might be more likely to forget the assessment when the patient has not spontaneously disclosed something about the violence, and that the therapist inadvertently conducts the assessment in a manner that discourages disclosure of violence.

When survivors of intimate partner violence are asked to predict the likelihood of future violence in their relationship within the subsequent year, they are accurate more often than not (Cattaneo et al., 2007). Thus, there is tremendous value in conveying your belief in the patient's intuition and good judgment about the relationship. As described later in this chapter, successful therapy with a patient who is experiencing relationship violence largely depends on the patient's trust in the therapist, and the more a therapist can do to convey that they believe the patient, are nonjudgmental, and will always prioritize the patient's goals over their own, the more likely it is that the patient will continue working with the therapist.

Mandated Disclosures

In many locations in the United States, most intimate partner violence that has already happened is insufficient to mandate reporting to any legal entities. However, there are some exceptions to that rule, which might vary based on location. If the partner violence was witnessed by children in the home, this might require a mandated disclosure to a state child protection agency. Violence perpetrated against an older adult or disabled adult might also result in mandated disclosure to an adult protection agency. Patients need to be informed about these mandated disclosure rules at the time that they consent to assessment or treatment. Typically, consent for treatment occurs before the therapist is aware of ongoing violence in the relationship. When the therapist learns of violence in the relationship and there are children living in the home, or the patient is disabled or an older adult, the therapist should remind the patient of the mandated disclosure rules and work collaboratively with them to disclose the violence to required agencies wherever possible. These disclosures should be accompanied by preparation of a safety plan for the patient, as it is possible that mandated disclosure (while well intended and legally required) might increase the risk for more violence. Best practices for making mandated disclosures include:

- informing the patient about the need to make a mandated disclosure, as well as provide them with details about why;
- discussing some possible outcomes of the mandated disclosure, ranging from the disclosure being minimized or ignored by the agency; being investigated by the agency but ultimately deemed to be without merit; being deemed to be a merited risk that requires changes for safety in the home; or some unanticipated alternative outcome;

- exploring the possibility of calling the reporting agency together;
- discussing whether it might be possible to anonymously discuss the nature of the violence without providing identifying information unless the agency deems that the situation merits reporting. Note that in some locations, anonymous consultations are possible, but not everywhere. Sometimes calling the agency back and connecting to a different agent results in different information about whether anonymous consultation is possible prior to formal disclosure (if mandated);
- officially reporting the incident to the required agency; and
- supporting the patient in navigating the aftermath of a mandated disclosure, including implementing components of their safety plan.

Sometimes mandated disclosures obliterate trust between the patient and the therapist. However, when navigated thoughtfully, with psychoeducation and with close attention to the emotional and logistical needs of the patient, mandated disclosures can increase trust in the therapeutic relationship.

Social Network Dynamics in the Context of Intimate Partner Violence

Survivors of intimate partner violence commonly experience a reduction in social support outside of their relationship following the introduction of violence into it. This sometimes occurs because the survivor may disclose the violence to someone in their support network, such as a friend or family member, who has an immediate (understandable) reaction of encouraging the patient to terminate the relationship. This dynamic happens in many relationships, even ones in which violence does not occur, after a partner discloses personal and negative details about the relationship to a loved one. To be supportive, family members will side with their loved one and, to provide support, actively disparage the partner. If the relationship continues, it is common for the partner to exert more secrecy about the nature of their conflict. For instance, your patient might say, "I already know that my mom doesn't like my boyfriend, so I can't really tell her about our fight. Chances are we will make up anyway, and if we do, she will just hate him more." Given that this dynamic can happen even with nonviolent relationship conflicts, it is possible that the pattern may become even more extreme in the context of violence.

In relationships characterized by unidirectional violence (from one partner to the other, but not in the other direction), the perpetrator of violence typically has a vested interest in promoting secrecy about their behavior. They recognize the potential for widespread negative consequences if other people learn about their abuse, including criminal charges being filed against them, other legal repercussions related to custody and divorce proceedings, negative social perceptions that might reduce their social standing (including career implications), and a greater risk that members of the social network will encourage their partner to leave the relationship. If the relationship ends, the perpetrator of violence may realize that their likelihood of procuring a new romantic partner may be reduced if others know about their abusive behavior. The stakes are high for these perpetrators of violence, which might motivate their attempts to encourage secrecy about the relationship. They might reinforce messages such as "We shouldn't air our dirty laundry" and "It's a violation of my trust/disrespectful for you to discuss our relationship with other people." The more that an abusive person can convince their partner to reduce or eliminate their social network, the more they can protect themselves from the significant consequences of their abuse.

Abusive partners commonly engage in controlling behaviors even during nonviolent periods in the relationship in order to diminish the quality and quantity of their partner's social network. People who engage in violence in romantic relationships might criticize their partner's family members, friends, colleagues, and acquaintances. They might also exhibit jealous behavior when their partner attempts to spend time with other people, which can increase the potential for more relationship violence. Given this frightening and exhausting dynamic, it might become easier for the partners of abusive people to reduce the amount of time that they spend with other people. People in the social network of a survivor of violence might fear the abusive partner and decide to back out of their friendship with the survivor. The ultimate consequence of this dynamic is that the survivor of violence may have few people in their lives to help them, including when they decide to leave the relationship. This reduced social circle further reinforces the perception (or aspects of the reality) of being trapped in the relationship, as the survivor of abuse may feel that they have nowhere to go if they leave their abusive partner.

Up to 51% of relationships with violence are characterized by bidirectional violence, in which both partners have physically harmed the other (Bates, 2016). A patient who is in such a relationship may be reluctant to disclose the mutual violence to their therapist for fear of negative judgment. The patient may also end up in a cycle of abuse where they feel further trapped in the relationship because of perceptions that they are partially or solely responsible for the violence. A patient in such a relationship may have thoughts such as, "I deserve this because of my behavior." Taking on an excessive degree of self-blame and self-diminishment may result in further polarization of beliefs about the partner as being high value.

Violence in relationships is often passed down in families. When children witness violence in their caregivers' relationships, they might perceive that violence is a common or even expected component of romantic partnerships. Survivors of violence may experience that their beliefs about violence are reaffirmed when they share details about their abuse with family members who react by normalizing or minimizing the experience. Such families might also invalidate a patient's PTSD symptoms by conveying that they are "making too big of a deal" of the violence or by explaining that their PTSD symptoms are a sign that the patient is "too sensitive."

The social dynamic of your patients cannot be ignored when they are experiencing intimate partner violence. Many of your patients in an abusive relationship will have a limited number of people to whom they can turn for support or safe haven. Other patients might be motivated to hide the nature of the violence in their relationship for fear that you will judge them and their partner, especially when friends and family have understandably engaged in such judgment. Still others might have limited insight into the fact that the violence is inappropriate because they have been exposed to violence in their caregivers' relationship from a young age. Patients who grew up in abusive families might find that their families invalidate their PTSD symptoms and even discourage their attendance in therapy. Given their tenuous social network, survivors of violence need a therapist who can serve as a nonjudgmental advocate to support them in achieving their goals for the relationship and other aspects of their lives, regardless of the direction that they ultimately choose to pursue.

Therapeutic Stance When Working With Survivors of Intimate Partner Violence

Survivors of intimate partner violence will likely hesitate to disclose details of their relationship due to complicated learning histories from opening up to others in the past. Patients may use their early sessions with a therapist to attempt to determine how much they can trust the therapist. As mentioned previously, including a standardized, formal assessment of relationship violence is one way to convey that the therapist is comfortable discussing this taboo topic and will neither overreact nor underreact to the information. Overreacting to a history of violence in a patient's relationship can be just as therapeutically harmful as underreacting. When the therapist has learned about violence in the relationship, it can help to assess how the *patient* feels about the violence rather than conveying the therapist's own perspective toward it. If the patient explicitly asks how the therapist views the violence, it may help to honestly convey to the patient that the therapist's opinion has no place in the patient's relationship, and what really matters is how the patient feels about the violence in their relationship. However, if a therapist is worried about a patient's imminent safety, making a safety plan becomes the number one priority (discussed next).

Whenever possible, it is best to convey a therapeutic stance that prioritizes therapeutic neutrality in terms of whether the therapist thinks that the patient should leave their romantic partner. If a therapist conveys that they think that the patient should leave their romantic partner, this disclosure can back a patient into a corner where they are forced to choose between staying with their partner or pleasing their therapist. In most cases, the therapist will lose that battle, and the patient's sense of safety in therapy may be damaged, which might prevent the patient from continuing in therapy.

Safety Plans for Survivors of Intimate Partner Violence

In any relationship with a history of violence, a safety plan offers an opportunity for your patient to anticipate a future episode in which they feel unsafe in the relationship. The National Domestic Violence Hotline (https://www.thehotline.org/) offers a wealth of resources to assist you and your patient in making a safety plan. The most basic plan includes preparing a bag for the patient to be ready to take at a moment's notice so that, if violence escalates, no packing is needed. The goal of this safety bag is to help the patient think through the essentials in their home that they will need and want to have at their disposal without having to return home if they leave in a hurry. This bag should include basic clothing items needed, necessary toiletries (e.g., contact lens solution and cases, a backup pair of glasses, shampoo, conditioner, body wash, toothbrush, toothpaste, dental floss, a backup mouth retainer, sanitary pads/tampons, etc.), backup medications where possible, an extra set of car keys, a pay-as-you-go mobile phone, a first aid kit, photocopies of essential legal documents (e.g., passport, driver's license, social security card, birth certificate), and potentially a cheap technology option for internet connectivity (i.e., a stripped-down laptop that can be purchased cheaply on sale). Patients also need to consider whether it is possible to secure credit cards that are independent from their partner so that the partner cannot turn off access to the credit if the patient needs it for gas, a hotel stay, and other emergency needs. Relationships characterized by physical abuse are often accompanied by financial abuse and control, so establishing a safety bag with the bare necessities can take a long time in those situations. It is important to attempt to store a safety bag where it will not be noticed by the abusive partner, as the partner's discovery of the bag can increase the risk of violence. The therapist should raise this possibility proactively with the patient, for instance by saying, *How can you put together this bag in a way that doesn't jeopardize your safety? Where can you store it that won't raise alarms? Are there things in the bag that we should remove because they will raise suspicion if discovered?*

A comprehensive safety plan includes consideration of where the patient could stay if violence escalates, as well as a plan for childcare and pet care if relevant. Many people remain in violent situations because they do not have great options for shelters that will allow children or pets. When a patient is in a crisis in which violence escalates, their problem-solving abilities may be reduced (typical of most emotional crises), which can make it harder to come up with solutions for finding shelter. Therefore, it can be essential to anticipate possible safe places to stay temporarily *before* the next crisis. It might also be essential to discuss safety related to lethal means and technology as part of a comprehensive safety plan. In particular, the patient can be encouraged to explore options to store lethal means safely before the next crisis and to ensure that they have a plan for turning off global positioning system (GPS) tracking on technology during the next crisis. Finally, the patient should explore local laws related to breaking rental leases in the context of intimate partner violence, as some locations have laws in place to protect survivors of abuse by allowing them to terminate a lease early.

Final Notes About Therapeutic Stance in Preparation for CBT for PTSD for Survivors of Intimate Partner Violence

After discussing the details of making a plan to promote safety, it can be difficult to resist the urge to encourage your patient to leave an unsafe relationship. If you attempt to convince your patient to prioritize their safety by leaving the relationship, it can backfire by forcing the patient to argue about the positive or necessary aspects of the relationship. This can drive a wedge in the therapeutic dynamic. A patient has a greater chance of feeling empowered to leave an unsafe relationship when they are free to make their own decisions and feel supported in their deliberations rather than feeling like they will disappoint their therapist if they decide to stay. If a patient decides to leave a relationship to avoid disappointing the therapist, the patient may blame the therapist for the decision in the future. If the patient plans to stay in a relationship despite fears that the therapist will be disappointed, they may feel shame about their decision and hide things from the therapist or cease therapy altogether.

Finally, abusive partners will commonly discourage therapy. The therapist should have explicit conversations with the patient about how the patient should share information about therapy with their partner. It can be helpful to assume that the abusive partner might somehow learn about the details of the therapy, and to always speak respectfully about them while still validating the patient's emotional experiences. If a therapist disparages the patient's partner, the partner may learn about this and further discourage the patient from attending therapy. The patient might benefit from practicing how to describe the therapy to the partner in a way that is honest and builds buy-in for continued therapy from the partner (versus making the partner perceive the therapy as a threat to relationship stability). If the patient's partner does not know about the therapy, the therapist might consider discussing what might happen if the partner finds out, and how they can collaboratively reduce the risk of that disclosure where possible (e.g., what happens if a bill from the health system arrives at the house and the partner sees it?)

Assessing Readiness to Begin CBT for PTSD in the Context of Intimate Partner Violence

Assessing readiness for CBT for PTSD is an ongoing process rather than a decision made at only one point in therapy. In most situations in which there is active violence in a romantic partnership, I strongly recommend waiting until the patient is in a safe environment before beginning CBT for PTSD. This is because CBT for PTSD can stir up difficult emotions that might make a patient feel more emotionally vulnerable. Coping with ongoing violence in the face of increased emotional vulnerability might create harm for the patient.

However, some patients present for CBT for PTSD when they are living in an actively violent relationship, have PTSD because of abuse from the relationship (or prior traumas), and the PTSD is interfering with the patient's confidence to leave the relationship. Remembering that (as discussed in Chapter 9) PTSD often significantly reduces a patient's beliefs about their power and control, when a patient is struggling with significant PTSD symptoms, it can be even harder than usual to feel capable of making a significant change, such as moving or ending a romantic partnership. In these cases, the patient and therapist should discuss the pros and cons of starting CBT while the patient is still in their relationship. This decision should be made *by* the patient rather than *for* the patient.

Trauma-Related Cognitions for Survivors of Intimate Partner Violence

For survivors of intimate partner violence, beliefs about self, others, and the world can shift dramatically and result in the maintenance of PTSD symptoms and of the relationship itself. Examples of negative beliefs about the self include "I am responsible for what happened" or "I deserve to be treated this way," whereas negative beliefs about other people include "Other partners would be even worse," and negative beliefs about the world include "There is nowhere safe from violence." These beliefs, when unaddressed, lead to decisions to stay in violent partnerships, risking further exposure to trauma.

Even when a violent relationship has ended, survivors of trauma struggle with beliefs about themselves that keep them stuck in misery. For example, a patient who is high achieving in their professional circle might be mortified about having been abused in the home, and after the relationship is over, they might prolong their pain by saying, "I should have known better than to be in this relationship" or "Other people like me would have left sooner." It is easy for survivors of violence to invalidate themselves by forgetting some of the legitimate reasons why they remained in the relationship. In these circumstances, it can be helpful to ask the patient to make a list of 10 reasons why it made perfect sense that they stayed in the relationship. Patients might counter with "But even my friends told me to leave," in which case it can be helpful to ask them to reflect on how there must have been many compelling reasons to stay at the time, in light of how other people tried to encourage them to leave.

If a patient has the belief that "I should have known better," it might be helpful to engage in a normalizing exercise by prompting the patient to take a perspective of a loved one in a violent relationship. For instance, the therapist might ask, *If your sibling was in a violent relationship and finally mustered the strength to leave, would your first thought be to blame them?* Typically, patients respond with, "Absolutely not, I would never think that!" In such cases, it can be helpful to ask the patient to make a list of 10 reasons why they should be held to higher standards than other people.

In Vivo Exposures for Survivors of Intimate Partner Violence

As with all *in vivo* exposures, it is essential to be clear on their goal prior to beginning. It can be common for survivors of intimate partner violence to be tempted to share details about their trauma with others, and it can be helpful to coach them on ensuring that the goal of the communication is about something that they must learn about themselves, as opposed to having a goal about how other people will react. For instance, if a patient is hoping that others will provide them with reassurance or treat them better, it might be helpful to discuss how this is a possible outcome, but that another possible outcome is that it will not elicit a healing response in another person, and could even elicit a harmful response. If the patient's goal is to learn about their ability to be confident in sharing the fact that they have survived violence, it might still be worth it for them to engage in such an *in vivo exposure* as long as the patient recognizes that the goal is not based on the reaction of the person receiving the information.

For some survivors of intimate partner violence, it can be helpful to do *in vivo* exposure exercises related to learning about stories of other people who have survived violence in their relationships. There are numerous websites where survivors of violence can share their stories online, and this might be a helpful exercise for some patients. For others, it can be helpful to watch media where a relationship is conveyed with power and control dynamics or violence. Some survivors might benefit from joining a support group as an *in vivo* exposure exercise, and there are many virtual and in-person options for such groups, depending on the patient's location.

Imaginal Exposure Considerations for Survivors of Intimate Partner Violence

In a desire to help other people understand the intensity of the trauma that they survived, some patients are tempted to share their imaginal exposure recordings with other people. We almost always strictly encourage patients to keep their recordings private. Even if the patient wants others to know what happened to them in general, it is rare that a loved one is prepared to emotionally handle the exact details of the trauma. Thus, while we generally strongly prefer that patients are positioned to make their own choices about *in vivo* exposures and the pacing of imaginal exposures (i.e., when to switch to hot spots, which hot spot to choose), we tend to directly instruct them not to share the imaginal exposure recordings with anyone.

Exposure to the Former Perpetrator of Violence

Survivors of intimate partner violence are sometimes in a unique position, relative to other trauma survivors, in terms of a need to have an ongoing relationship with the perpetrator of violence. This is particularly relevant when children are involved and shared custody arrangements require coparenting. It can also be relevant related to court proceedings for the dissolution of marriage or division of assets. Part of the goal of CBT for PTSD is supporting the patient to feel as self-confident as possible in interactions with the perpetrator when necessary. This includes continuing to have safety at the top of the priority list, relying on mediators for communication as possible, and building an emotional distress tolerance plan to help the patient recover from encounters with the perpetrator. Finally, it can be helpful to role-play some prepared verbal responses if the perpetrator engages in conversation topics that the patient wants to avoid. For instance, the therapist might work with the patient to redirect the conversation back to a necessary topic (e.g., "We really just need to figure out the drop-off plans for this weekend") or to stop the conversation in its tracks through active ignoring or by establishing a boundary ("If you do not stop contacting me, I'm going to have to file for a protective order") and reinforcing that boundary ("Because you contacted me again, I am filing a protective order").

Summary

In this chapter, I reviewed the cycle of abuse that maintains violence in some relationships, as well as social dynamics that are relevant to the context of providing CBT for PTSD. I discussed the therapeutic stance in CBT for PTSD, navigating mandated disclosures, and maintaining a focus on safety as needed. I discussed core considerations in determining patients' readiness for CBT for PTSD. I also reviewed common trauma-related cognitions that emerge in the context of intimate partner violence, as well as some strategies to support patients in processing the cognitions in order to heal. Finally, I discussed considerations for *in vivo* and imaginal exposures, and supporting patients through future encounters with their perpetrators.

12 Navigating the Legal System in PTSD Treatment

Intersections With the Legal System Following Trauma

Having some knowledge of the local legal context facilitates the provision of high-quality CBT for PTSD. In this chapter, I discuss some high-level considerations about the intersection of trauma and the legal system to support therapists in their provision of CBT. While therapists do not need to become experts in legal considerations, they are best able to advocate for and help prepare their patients for legal involvement following trauma exposure if they have some understanding of the local legal processes that their patients may encounter.

Involvement in the Legal System and the Impact on PTSD Symptoms

There have been a variety of reports that explored involvement in the legal system and the impact on PTSD symptoms, particularly because of inaccurate perceptions that PTSD symptoms are motivated by attempts to seek compensation following trauma exposure. However, when patients with no compensation, settled compensation, and ongoing compensation are compared on demographic and psychopathology measures, there are no differences between the groups, and this lack of differences is maintained at 6-month follow-up (Bryant & Harvey, 2003). Perhaps not surprisingly, people who never initiated compensation proceedings were less likely to meet criteria for PTSD than patients with settled or ongoing compensation (Bryant & Harvey, 2003). Thus, patients who present for treatment for PTSD have a greater chance of having some involvement in the legal system, which makes it important for therapists to know a bit about their local context for court involvement.

Criminal and Civil Cases

Depending on the nature of the trauma, your patients might be involved in criminal, civil, or both types of cases related to the trauma. Their involvement might include everything from having to testify against a perpetrator, providing statements to police and investigators, being implicated in the aftermath of a trauma legally as a defendant, or attending court proceedings to learn of the outcomes. It is essential to understand the legal involvement of your patient before they commence CBT for PTSD, both related to the index trauma and unrelated. It can be helpful to assess their understanding of the anticipated timeline for decisions related to ongoing legal involvement, noting that this timeline is subject to change at the whim of the court. In addition, it can be helpful to understand whether the patient is anticipating that a civil lawsuit will follow a criminal lawsuit, as relevant, to inform the timeline of ongoing legal battles. For patients who are represented by a lawyer, it might be helpful to request clarification about how, if at all, the mental health treatment of the patient could become relevant to the court proceedings. Even in circumstances in which the patient and their lawyer suspect that treatment is unlikely to have relevance for the case, it is essential to document treatment with an expectation that it will be potentially subpoenaed for the ongoing legal proceedings at some point in the future. In some cases, records are subpoenaed years after the treatment is concluded, and the therapist's documentation will be essential for the therapist to refresh their memory about the case. For this reason, documentation should be thorough to satisfy billing requirements as well as to provide a summary to understand the treatment focus, but it should not include unnecessary details that could become part of a future trial. For instance, the therapist should document what type of *in vivo* or imaginal exposure homework was assigned but does not need to share each detail of the imaginal exposure script beyond the type of the index trauma as it relates to the provision of a PTSD diagnosis (contingent on a criterion A trauma exposure).

It is also helpful to understand the patient's involvement in legal battles that are not directly related to the trauma. Patients who are on house arrest will have fewer options for *in vivo* exposure practice and might not have a private space to listen to their imaginal exposure recordings for homework. If a patient is anticipating incarceration, it might not be ideal to start CBT for PTSD if you suspect that treatment will be interrupted before progress can be achieved (this is discussed in more detail later in this chapter). Patients who are under another form of surveillance, such as being out on probation or on parole, might also have limited options in terms of their associates or travel options. In some cases, it might be helpful (with the patient's permission) to collaborate with a parole/probation officer to obtain permission for the patient to engage in homework exercises for CBT for PTSD or to come to sessions more frequently to help them work through the distress of imaginal exposures more quickly. Prior to beginning CBT for PTSD, it is very helpful to understand your patient's current legal involvement so you can plan treatment appropriately.

Sharing Stories With Police and Investigators

As described in Chapter 6 on imaginal exposures, patients commonly must share details of their trauma numerous times before coming to CBT for PTSD. They might have had to give a statement to police when the initial trauma happened, which might need to be repeated multiple times later to different police officers or investigators. They might have had to share their story with a medical professional in the context of receiving care following exposure to a trauma, as could be the case with a rape kit. For cases that involve ongoing legal entanglements, the patient might expect to need to repeat the description of the trauma on many more occasions, even if they would prefer for a legal case not to happen. When starting CBT for PTSD, it is essential to recognize that patients may have had a wide range of experiences when they shared their story previously, ranging from disinterest to doubt and denial, defensiveness, and validation. It can be helpful to learn about the patient's prior experiences in sharing their trauma narrative with other people to help understand how it might be most helpful for you to respond as you start to work together.

As discussed in Chapter 6, the fact that a patient has told their story numerous times, and potentially must continue to do so, can make it challenging for them to engage in imaginal exposure even when it is clinically indicated. It can be helpful to remind the patient that imaginal exposure provides an opportunity to feel whatever they need to feel in retelling their story, and to give themselves permission to open up emotionally during the revisiting process. This is often in stark contrast to the emotionally shut-down recounting that sometimes happens in a legal setting, when patients muster all their strength to stifle emotional expression as they share the most horrible events of their lives.

Unpredictability of the Court System

The court system can be extremely unpredictable, which increases anxiety for patients with PTSD. Most of my patients with a court date found that the trial was ultimately delayed. Explanations for why a court date is delayed run the gamut from scheduling conflicts, preparation time delays, a witness who is unable to be located or who needs to have the date postponed, or that the judge needs additional time to review relevant documentation. For my patients who are newer to legal involvement, it can be very surprising and discouraging when a court date is delayed. This is especially true when a patient has been rallying their psychological state to prepare for that date. Thus, it can be helpful to inform patients about this possibility when you assess their current legal status.

Another source of unpredictability in the legal system is how and when decisions are made related to the incarceration and release of perpetrators. Some of my patients have survived grisly traumas where they were certain that the perpetrator would be found guilty or would never be released from prison, only to find that a technicality or other surprising outcome resulted in the release of the perpetrator. This unpredictability can be terrifying for survivors of PTSD, who may be fearful about the potential for retaliation.

A third scenario of unpredictability in the legal system is related to perpetrators who are unable to be located and arrested at all. Sometimes patients are understandably surprised at how it is possible for the perpetrator to evade the law. In these circumstances, it is common for the trauma survivor with PTSD to feel nervous about staying at their residence or taking routes known to the perpetrator. Some patients avoid taking public transit out of fear that they could run into the perpetrator at any stop. These fears are not necessarily irrational, but they have a major impact on decisions about the relative safety or danger of certain CBT practices for PTSD, such as *in vivo* exposure practices.

Readiness for CBT for PTSD in the Context of Legal Involvement

If legal proceedings related to an index trauma are likely to resolve soon, it may not make sense to begin CBT for PTSD until the legal battles have concluded. Deciding to delay CBT for PTSD until a trial is concluded is sensible when there is a possibility that treatment might stir up difficult emotions that the patient would like to avoid for the moment. However, the unpredictability of court proceedings makes it challenging to perfectly plan treatment to avoid this possibility. Even with the best intentions of waiting until legal matters are resolved, with unexpected delays in court dates or changes in the status of the freedom of a trauma perpetrator, the CBT therapist needs to be willing to be flexible in treatment to respond to changing dynamics. That can include collaboratively deciding with the patient that it makes sense to delay treatment, pause it, or change the intensity of the treatment sessions in some meaningful way until the legal battle is resolved.

For some patients, the legal consequences of their trauma will not resolve in their lifetime. In these cases, it is essential to support the patient in deciding on the pros and cons of starting or continuing in CBT for PTSD. One of the major pros of staying the course and seeing CBT for PTSD through is that the patient may feel more confident about their emotion regulation ability during the court proceedings if they have emotionally processed the trauma via CBT. One of the major cons of proceeding with CBT for PTSD, however, is that it may stir up difficult emotions and make the court dates and sessions even more difficult for the patient to endure. However, most patients with PTSD have regular, intrusive memories about the trauma that already make it challenging for them to function effectively in court. It is possible that CBT will teach them skills to feel better prepared for court.

Social Support to Navigate Legal Proceedings

Anyone going through lengthy court proceedings would benefit from social support. As patients with PTSD proceed through CBT, some will benefit from *in vivo* exposures focused on growing their social network in preparation for getting the support that they will need for court and other aspects of their lives. Patients might feel more comfortable going to court when they have people who can come with them. For patients who are socially isolated, there may be circumstances where it is advantageous for the therapist to join the patient at a court hearing (obviously only at the request of the patient and never in the absence of advance permission from them).

CBT therapists need to maintain the highest ethical standards to always protect professional boundaries, including if they decide to accompany a patient to a court date. This means that the patient and therapist should proactively discuss the following:

- How the therapist should identify themselves when asked (i.e., is the patient OK with the therapist disclosing that they are presenting to court to support their patient?)
- That the CBT therapist is accompanying the patient in a professional role to provide support, but that it will not change the dynamic of their professional arrangement
- The number of times that the therapist can realistically plan to join the patient, especially given that court dates are frequently moved with little notice and the therapist might not be able to set aside multiple days for attendance at a trial
- That the goal is to continue growing the patient's network of support so they have folks that they can trust to support them in similar situations in the future, which will be part of the focus of CBT

It goes without saying that there is no expectation that CBT therapists join their patients in court. Even when therapists wish that they had the flexibility in their schedule to join, they still might be unable to do so. Protecting time to attend a court hearing can easily absorb half to a full day of time in a therapist's schedule. This is not practical for most therapists in most settings. However, when it is practical and comfortable for the therapist, and when there is no risk of an ethical violation, it can be extremely rewarding for the patient to have the support of their therapist in court.

Distress Tolerance Plan for After a Court Proceeding

As legal changes approach, it can be helpful for patients to anticipate that they will feel more emotionally raw around the time of court hearings or changes in legal status. A CBT therapist can help their patient by generating a distress tolerance plan to help them survive extremely upsetting news during the legal battle. The idea behind a distress tolerance plan is to proactively anticipate what types of strategies might be helpful for reducing emotional intensity and securing necessary components of the plan before they are needed. If the patient finds certain sensory stimuli very soothing, they might benefit from gathering those stimuli in advance so that they will have them when upset. Alternatively, if the patient would find it helpful to make social plans after a court date or to plan to take themselves to a special location to self-soothe, the CBT therapist can support the patient in planning for these options.

Securing a Protective Order/Restraining Order

Some patients might come to therapy with a desire to seek a protective order to prevent a perpetrator of their trauma from contacting them or coming into close proximity of them. The process for securing a protective order can be complicated and prolonged even in situations where it might appear obvious that an order would be granted. There are a few considerations that a CBT therapist should make to support their patient in this process.

Documentation Is Key

Keeping close documentation of all relevant information is essential for successfully receiving a protective order. Usually, this begins with filing a police report, which might need to be repeated more than once to build a case to support the order. Patients should hold onto documentation of all inappropriate communications that were written, emailed, or texted to them from the perpetrator, and patients should also have a call log of incoming/missed calls or other attempts at contact from the perpetrator. Voicemails should be saved, and inappropriate or threatening communications that happen in person or over the phone should be described in writing by the patient, along with a log of what was said and when. The patient should know their local laws for recording without the permission of the perpetrator and, where legal, consider recording communications that occur. The patient should seek legal advice on this, and on whether they should attempt to block the perpetrator from communication versus allowing the perpetrator to continue contacting them to record the persistence of the contact attempts (as well as inappropriate text messages, emails, or voicemails).

Coping With Invalidation

For some people who seek a protective order, the experience can be extremely invalidating. In the process of filing a police report, patients might find that their report is not taken seriously, and they might even be actively discouraged from filing. In some locations, a protective order will not be granted in the absence of police involvement or a police report, so patients should be encouraged to be persistent even in the face of invalidation. CBT therapists can help the patient to identify cope-ahead statements to manage the distress of invalidation, as well as strategies to support assertive communication to make the requests repeatedly and in a respectful but determined manner.

Preparing to See the Perpetrator in Court

If a protective order is considered in a court, it is possible that the patient will have to be at court with the perpetrator. They may have to verbalize why they are making the request and back up the evidence that they present in court. Some courts will allow a court advocate to be present in these hearings, but not all provide them. The CBT therapist can support the patient in role-playing how they want to engage with the perpetrator. For instance, the therapist and patient can discuss how the patient will behave if they see the perpetrator in the hall before court or outside the courthouse. They might also need to come up with some cope-ahead statements to muster the courage to see the process through in the face of fear of seeing the perpetrator.

Preparing for a Protective Order to Be Denied

Even when patients do everything in their power to secure a protective order and have sufficient documentation to support that, they are not in control of the ultimate outcome. In some cases, patients are denied protective orders even when it would seem obvious to the therapist and the patient that a protective order is in the best interest of the safety of everyone involved. CBT therapists should have a problem-solving conversation with the patient in advance about what to do if a protective order is denied.

Preparing for Violations of Orders

When a protective order is granted, the perpetrator will sometimes violate it. I have worked with patients where a violation of the order happened almost immediately after it was granted. The patient would benefit from problem solving in advance on what to do if that occurs, who to contact, and how to prioritize and protect their safety.

Preparing for Need to Renew Orders

In many locations, protective orders are temporary and need to be renewed every few years. This is an emotionally difficult experience for patients who may feel like the wound of their trauma is reopened each time they have to advocate for protection from the perpetrator. Note that protective orders sometimes need to be renewed even if an order is violated (resulting in additional legal trouble). The CBT therapist can support the patient in viewing the protective order as a temporary arrangement that will allow the patient to get distance from the perpetrator, but that will not be permanent.

Incarceration of the Perpetrator

When a patient has a protective order, in some cases they will be informed if the perpetrator has become incarcerated. This is particularly relevant when the perpetrator violates the protective order, is not immediately located, and then later becomes incarcerated. In such circumstances, the patient may also be informed when the perpetrator will be released from incarceration. The CBT therapist can support the patient in requesting communication from the detective to whom they were assigned (as relevant) about this information if it is helpful for them.

Wariness of People Who Take Advantage of Trauma Survivors to "Help" Them

When a person experiences a trauma, they can be in a vulnerable state of mind as they recover. When a person is involved in a legal battle while they recover from a trauma, their vulnerability is even more intense. This can be a time when other people might seek to take advantage of them. It can be helpful for the therapist to assess changes in the patient's support system to gather information about this possibility. One example that I have seen repeatedly in my practice are situations where a new person moves into the patient's home under the guise of "helping" the patient to feel safer, while simultaneously taking advantage of the patient's generosity or even potentially increasing conflict in the home. Patients can feel stuck in these situations because they might worry that others will not take them seriously if they have had two violent or untrustworthy people in their lives. Therefore, providing normalizing around these experiences in the service of supporting the patient in self-advocacy can be an important role for a CBT therapist.

Custody and Disability Determinations

A final challenging legal consideration while providing CBT for PTSD is related to custody arrangements and disability determinations. The patient and CBT therapist should clarify at the beginning of treatment whether the patient has goals related to therapy for support in a custody battle or determination of disability. The therapist should clarify that the goal in their treatment is *not* to be in a court of law and instead to help the patient to heal emotionally from their trauma as needed. This is particularly relevant in the context of imaginal exposure; the goal of exposure is not to make a memory more accurate or to increase confidence about a memory. If patients hope that their treatment will offer them additional credibility in their court proceedings, it can be helpful to remind them about the importance of CBT being reserved for healing. Patients in these situations might benefit from a referral to a legal expert, such as a forensic psychologist, to support them in documenting what is needed for a custody arrangement or disability determination. In this way, the focus of therapy can remain on wellness without the distraction of worrying about the impact of healing (or struggling emotionally) on the legal battle.

Summary

In this chapter, I discussed considerations for CBT therapists when their patients are embroiled in legal battles either as a direct result of their trauma or for unrelated reasons. First, I provided an overview of the importance of assessing legal involvement before treatment begins. Second, I discussed readiness for CBT based on the status of legal battles. Third, I discussed protective orders and key considerations for CBT therapists who support patients with PTSD in procuring this option. Finally, I briefly covered the difference between CBT for PTSD and psychological assessments that are helpful for custody or disability determinations.

13 Training Supervisees in Evidence-Based Practices for PTSD

There is wide recognition that trauma can affect psychological health in myriad ways, and many therapists who do not view themselves as experts in treating PTSD are attending to trauma in their clinical work. However, as discussed in Chapter 1, most trauma survivors do not meet the criteria for PTSD, and when a therapist is attempting to provide treatment for PTSD for the first time, it can be overwhelming. Informal case consultation and formal supervision are the optimal ways to ensure that therapists who are new to providing CBT for PTSD have the support that they need.

The Frame of Supervision

Framing supervision in a manner that parallels the framing of a CBT session can support trainees in learning how to structure their time with patients effectively. This can include starting supervision with a mood check, which can either be quantitative (i.e., 0–10, where 10 is the best mood ever and 0 is the worst) or qualitative. Just like CBT sessions with patients, CBT supervision benefits from a bridge from the prior supervision to refresh the supervisor and the trainee on what was discussed the previous week. Then the supervisor might begin by reviewing any goals that the trainee intended to complete between supervisions, and then asking the trainee for their agenda. Agendas should ideally be driven by the trainee except in rare circumstances, where the supervisor has an urgent issue that needs to be discussed before the trainee's items, such as a concern about safety or feedback that needs to be prioritized (e.g., an end-of-year evaluation). After all items on the agenda are completed, it is helpful to leave time for feedback so that the trainee can share their sense of how supervision is going, what is helpful, and what could be more helpful in the future.

Another critical piece to the framing of supervision for CBT for PTSD is the use of audio- or videotape reviews of sessions. Recording CBT for PTSD therapy sessions provides the best way for trainees to improve. There is no substitute for the value of recorded sessions for therapists who strongly desire to improve their skills. Therapists who have already received training in general CBT will likely have had a lot of experience with recording their therapy sessions, but therapists who are new to CBT might never have had experience with this.

Recording sessions can be extremely vulnerable for therapists who are eager to do a good job and who might feel intimated about receiving feedback from a more experienced supervisor. Because recording sessions can be anxiety provoking, some therapists avoid it at all costs, which strips them of a valuable learning opportunity. Other therapists will pitch it to patients in a manner that makes the patient very unlikely to agree to the recording. Not all patients will feel comfortable consenting to be recorded, but I often find that the way that we describe the rationale of the recording dictates the likelihood that a patient will agree.

When a trainee asks a patient to consider signing a consent form for recording therapy sessions, I often coach them to reiterate a few key points to the patient:

- The goal of the recording is to make sure that the therapist is delivering the treatment in the highest-quality manner possible.
- The supervisor, identified by name, will be watching or listening to the recording with more of a focus on what the therapist is saying and doing, than what the patient is saying and doing.
- Having an extra perspective from a trained professional can generate additional treatment ideas to ensure that the patient receives the best treatment possible.
- Most patients are nervous about it at first but tend to notice that after some time, they forget the recording is happening.

Most patients are willing to provide consent for their sessions to be observed with this rationale, especially because they are eager to get better. When patients do provide permission to record the session, note that this typically means that the therapist is recording the session using a clinic device, and the patient is usually audio-recording the session on their own personal device to listen to between sessions. This parallel process in CBT for PTSD helps to reduce discomfort about the recording of sessions.

Supporting the Therapist Who Is New to CBT for PTSD

Remember that when we help our patients with processing an imaginal exposure, we begin processing with warmth and encouragement; the same approach is helpful in supervision. Other than in rare circumstances of egregious misconduct, there are always details about sessions that can be celebrated to acknowledge a therapist's hard work. It is essential to make sure that you acknowledge what you observed that was encouraging, helpful, appropriate, and insightful about the way that they structured the sessions.

All therapists who are new to CBT for PTSD will have growth areas. I like to choose 1–3 growth areas to prioritize each supervision, even if many more were observed in each session. I will never forget a supervision session with my supervisor who had a multiple-page list of everything that I did in the session that should/could be changed for the future. When the supervisor was about halfway through the list, I was unsure whether to start crying at my ineptitude or laughing at the ridiculousness of the length (and specificity) of the feedback. At a certain point, my brain was no longer able to take in the feedback, and my learning was limited. I have no doubt that the supervisor's feedback was spot on, but I found it extremely difficult to watch my supervisor read a list of everything that I did wrong in a single session, without pausing, for what felt like an eternity. I remember walking away from the supervision with the realization that to be responsive to the feedback, I would have to try to do just about everything differently! It felt like an impossible task, even though I knew that the supervisor was right that I needed a great deal of improvement.

This lesson sticks with me many years later, and I try to practice what we aim for in exposure therapy: sufficient emotional engagement to promote new learning, but not such extreme upset that learning is not possible. Genuine feedback about improvement can be vulnerable for therapists, especially when they are already on edge because of the emotionally uncomfortable content that is the focus of CBT for PTSD. As supervisors, we must remember that our trainees are in a vulnerable position, and our feedback should be targeted and prioritized in terms of what is most essential, letting more nitpicky feedback wait until a later supervision. In supervision, as in therapy, even when we miss an opportunity to address a topic, the opportunity will present itself again in the future. By cheerleading our trainees' strengths, providing them with critical feedback, and holding back on nitpicking, we are helping to boost our trainees' confidence and skill simultaneously.

Common Mistakes by Therapists Who Are Newer to CBT for PTSD

Many therapists who are newer to providing CBT for PTSD will fall into predictable types of mistakes that become easy to catch the more experience that you have with supervision. In the following, I review some common examples of those mistakes and provide suggestions about how you can help a trainee to get unstuck.

Tendency to Fragilize

Patients with PTSD have strong emotional reactions to reminders of the trauma but this should not be mistaken for fragility. Sometimes, to protect their patients, therapists newer to CBT for PTSD worry about digging too deeply into their trauma, saying things that will make patients more upset, or encouraging patients to do things that will set them back. The tendency to fragilize patients with PTSD is sometimes inadvertently reinforced by the patients' own perspective of themselves, given that many patients with PTSD feel disempowered and out of control. To be optimally helpful in CBT for PTSD, therapists need to take the perspective that their patients can handle a great deal emotionally, and that there are few well-intentioned things that a therapist can say or do in the context of CBT for PTSD that will objectively worsen patients' suffering.

If you notice that a trainee is walking on eggshells around their patient or fragilizing them in some way, it can be helpful to explore the cognitions that are underlying these behaviors. It might help to pause the tape in supervision and ask the trainee to do a cognitive model with you where they describe what they were thinking, physically feeling, and tempted to do when they engaged in behaviors that conveyed fragilizing the patient. Commonly, fragilizing interpretations are not obvious to new therapists until they are discussed explicitly. It can be helpful to remind the trainee about the importance of trusting in the patient's strengths and skills so that the patient starts to recognize their value as well.

Common Mistakes by Therapists Who Are New to Imaginal Exposure

As mentioned in Chapter 6, imaginal exposure can be an intimidating therapeutic technique until CBT therapists have seen the benefit of the procedure. There are several common mistakes that new CBT therapists make when they start engaging in imaginal exposure.

Assuming That Any Emotional Activation Is Overengagement

Imaginal exposures are emotionally evocative by design. When done correctly, patients commonly emote intense emotional experiences, including crying, as they revisit their trauma memory. Experiencing strong emotions allows emotional healing and new learning to occur. However, when therapists are new to imaginal exposure, it is easy to confuse a patient's emoting with overengagement. If the therapist incorrectly assumes that the patient needs help in calming down during the imaginal exposure, the therapist runs the risk of interfering with the healing process. Even if a patient is communicating that their SUDs are maxed out (e.g., 100 out of 100), this does not necessarily mean that the process is off base. Revisiting a trauma memory is painful, and we must coach our trainees to be willing to witness the pain of patients as they work through it.

If a trainee is misinterpreting emotional activation as overengagement, it can be helpful to review those portions of the tape together. Sometimes, when the trainee can view the session in a more objective manner (when they are out of the "hot seat" of directing the CBT session), they immediately realize that the patient was appropriately engaged as opposed to overengaged. It might also help to discuss what you would see if the patient were overengaged (i.e., sobbing hysterically, unable to articulate the story from distress, threatening violence against the therapist because they are upset, etc.). Sometimes it can help to show your trainee tapes of your own clients (with your clients' permission, which I often request for training purposes) to demonstrate how emotionally evocative an early exposure is, and then how nonevocative it is later in treatment. Finally, it might help to brainstorm a list of ways that the trainee can become more aware of what is happening in the room in the presence of strong emotions, as well as to roleplay how they might like to respond if overengagement happens as opposed to being in the presence of expected emotional engagement.

Delaying the Start of Exposures

New trainees will often propose adding more sessions before the patient begins *in vivo* or imaginal exposure practice. Sometimes trainees propose to delay the start of exposures because they feel that the patient is not quite ready; for example, perhaps they feel that the patient does not yet have sufficient buy-in or that psychoeducation needs to be repeated. Sometimes the trainee is worried that a patient will become too distressed by doing an exposure, and therefore they might propose to delay it. It is best to base a decision about risk on objective data; for instance, if the patient recently engaged in self-harm or had a suicide attempt, delaying the start of exposures is very appropriate. Conversely, it is not appropriate to delay exposures because of the risk that they could be too upsetting for the patient.

Delaying exposures tends to backfire. It adds to their mystery and threat level for patients. Exposures become a nebulous, terrifying prospect, and patients sometimes drop out of therapy before exposures begin for this reason. Exposures often go well initially, and if the exposure had been delayed, then the trainee and patient would have wasted precious time that could have been spent moving toward recovery from PTSD. If a patient makes a request to delay, the trainee should honor that request, as the number one priority in CBT for PTSD is uplifting patients' autonomy and supporting their empowerment. In almost all cases, the suggestion to delay exposures is initiated by the therapist (not the patient), and the therapist should fight the urge to delay exposures unless there is a strong clinical reason to do so.

Interrupting

Imaginal exposures are a cognitively and emotionally demanding task. Some newer therapists are too distracting during the process, or their questions are too wordy, and they take the patient out of the immersive experience. The goal of the CBT therapist is to balance warmth and validation for the patient with staying out of the patient's way.

If your trainee is engaging in distracting behaviors, it can be helpful for them to watch those segments of the recording and to report back to you about what they observe. Sometimes, therapists are distracting to their patients because they are not prepared enough. They might be shuffling papers around, finding a pen, or moving a clock so that they can see it. These behaviors are easy to shape as they simply require supporting the trainee in getting more prepared before the exposure. In other cases, therapists are using words of encouragement too frequently to help metaphorically "hold the patient's hand" through the process. Too much encouragement during imaginal exposure prevents the patient from achieving immersion in their memory. In such cases, it can be helpful to show tape where the patient is having a hard time with engaging in the retelling immediately after one of these words of encouragement and asking the trainee for their observations about that segment. Finally, some therapists ask questions that are confusing or too lengthy, and they diminish the experience for the patient. You can coach your trainee to write down each question in advance to help make sure that it is worth asking and pithy.

Not Being Present Enough

Some trainees are terrified of interrupting the imaginal exposure practice and cope with that by saying very little throughout. It can be helpful to remind trainees that we want the patient to sense that we are in the room with them during their recounting and are able to help if they need us. Encouraging the trainee to vocalize some brief words of encouragement can help to make their presence more obvious during the exercise. Sometimes I coach trainees to say a word of encouragement immediately after requesting a SUDs rating to reduce the disruption as much as possible but still demonstrate warmth and validation for the patient.

Common Mistakes for Therapists Who Are New to Processing Following an Exposure

Processing exposures is unusual territory for many CBT therapists, particularly for processing of imaginal exposures. Processing tends to be less directive, and it is hard to prepare trainees for what to say during processing because it completely depends on the needs of the patient. The lack of structure is sometimes nerve-wracking for CBT therapists who might feel more comfortable providing psychoeducation or explaining how to do a task. In this section, I discuss common challenges that new CBT trainees experience when supporting their patients with processing and how to work through these challenges.

Taking the Lead When They Should Trust the Patient's Process

Processing an imaginal exposure is optimal when the patient takes the lead. New trainees are sometimes intimidated by the silence that can come up while a patient is cognitively working through the impact of a trauma, and they might attempt to fill the silence with a directive question. It is best to coach trainees to take a relaxed approach to processing, with a laser focus on what the patient is saying and how they are saying it. The best processing happens when the therapist is engaged in extremely mindful observation of the patient. This allows the therapist to get out of their own head, drop any preplanned questions, and focus on what is important for the patient to discuss. Only when the patient's initial reaction to the exposure runs out of steam is it appropriate for the therapist to ask more targeted questions, and even then they should limit the number of questions to 1–3 core domains.

As the CBT therapist is watching a patient do an exposure, they likely have dozens of potential questions to ask the patient. It can help to coach the therapist to think about marking the top 3 most important questions with stars and to only ask those 3 questions if the patient has run out of natural reactions to the exposure. Whatever questions the therapist cannot get to during this round of processing will be possible topics of conversation in future sessions.

Defaulting to Psychoeducation

When new CBT therapists get nervous that they do not know what to say, they sometimes cope with that anxiety by shifting gears into an area where they feel competent: didactics. Whenever a trainee has shifted into psychoeducation mode in processing, it can help to understand what motivated that shift. Occasionally, providing psychoeducation during processing is necessary and helpful. More commonly, psychoeducation results in reduced emotional expression in the session as the patient and therapist engage in an analytical discussion that is focused on logic as opposed to emotions. As the trainee watches their tapes back, it can be helpful to coach them to attend to the affect intensity in the session after they have shifted into psychoeducation, and to ask them what they might do differently the next time that they do not know what to say. I often like to model to my trainees the power of pausing in a therapy session and noting, *This is so important – let me think for a moment.* Trainees should be assuaged that silence in processing can be a sign that the patient is having important reflections and allowing for new learning to happen, and that this should not be rushed.

Rushing to Get to Healing

A new CBT therapist will sometimes have a strong hunch about what cognitions are contributing the most to their patients being stuck in suffering with PTSD. Sometimes our instincts as therapists are correct, and often we are mistaken when we do not yet have the full story. It is important for CBT therapists to be willing to not know for sure what changes will need to happen for a patient to heal from their PTSD. New therapists sometimes rush the process and might put pressure on themselves and the patient to resolve trauma cognitions. You might notice that this happens when your trainee tries to argue with a patient about how they should see things instead or tries to convince them of something that they had not yet considered. Very often, these well-intentioned attempts at rushing the process can feel invalidating to the patient. Thus, rather than asking leading questions or coaching the patient to see a cognition differently, supervisors can coach trainees to provide more open-ended follow-ups. For instance, say, *You said that you carry just as much blame for this as the person who assaulted you. Tell me more about that.* The supervisor might roleplay this with the trainee to help the trainee in taking a less directive approach to processing.

Summary

In this chapter, I discussed how to support trainees who are new to learning CBT for PTSD. I discussed how to frame supervision for maximal benefit, as well as how to balance encouragement with scaffolding constructive feedback. I also reviewed some of the common mistakes made by trainees when they first implement CBT for PTSD, including fragilizing patients, delaying the start of exposures, and rushing the process. Finally, I provided suggestions for supervisors to use when guiding newer therapists to address these common mistakes.

14 Implementing Evidence-Based Treatments for PTSD in the Community

Community mental health centers see significantly higher rates of PTSD compared to the general community. In our research in Philadelphia, over half (58.2%) of patients treated in community mental health centers screened above the clinical cutoff for probable PTSD on the Post-traumatic Diagnostic Scale for DSM-5 (PDS-5) (Pincus et al., 2022). Sometimes there is a question about appropriateness for evidence-based treatments in community mental health, given that comorbidity is the norm rather than the exception. However, in our own research, 100% of patients with PTSD in community mental health were deemed good candidates for PE therapy (Pincus et al., 2022) by their community clinician. When PE is administered in community clinics, patient outcomes are equivalent to specialty behavioral healthcare (Foa et al., 2005). Nevertheless, our team at the Center for the Treatment and Study of Anxiety have been implementing PE in the community in Philadelphia for over a decade and have learned some important considerations to ensure success for patients and clinicians.

Assessment

Community clinicians must have access to quick and reliable screening and assessment tools to confirm PTSD diagnoses. When PE was initially implemented in community mental health in Philadelphia, some of the clinicians had difficulty in identifying cases for PE because they were not familiar with the PTSD diagnosis. To address this, the Center for the Treatment and Study of Anxiety started offering a brief workshop just on assessment of PTSD in addition to their 4-day PE workshop. Once clinicians became more comfortable with implementing brief screenings and assessments for PTSD, more of their patients were deemed to be possible candidates for CBT for PTSD. In our community project, we typically train clinicians to use the Posttraumatic Diagnostic Scale for DSM-5 (PDS-5; Foa, McLean, Zang, Zhong, Powers, et al., 2016) because it includes the identification of the index trauma as well as assessment of PTSD severity. It can be helpful to follow this self-report measure with an interview, such as the PTSD Symptom Scale-Interview for DSM-5 (PSSI-5) (Foa, McLean, Zang, Zhong, Rauch, et al., 2016) to help the patient with questions that they have about differentiating symptoms and making sure that the symptoms that they are reporting are attributable to the index trauma.

Readiness for PE in Community Settings

In earlier chapters, I discussed readiness for PE as it related to intimate partner violence (Chapter 11) and in the context of legal involvement (Chapter 12). When thinking about readiness for PE in community settings, there are some common challenges that emerge that are common sources of questions for community therapists. One example is working with patients who have limited financial resources and multiple psychosocial stressors. A patient is unlikely to benefit from any therapy when their basic needs are unmet; working closely with a case manager to ensure that the patient has sufficient food and a safe place to live might be necessary before beginning the emotionally demanding work of CBT for PTSD. Another example is when a patient lives in a neighborhood stricken by gun violence and the therapist and patient need to make a determination about whether the patient is in a position of relative safety to begin therapy. In this case, the CBT therapist and the patient should have a conversation about the pros and cons of doing trauma-focused therapy. The pros include the possibility that PTSD symptoms will improve, which could reduce functional impairment and create new opportunities for the patient to consider building a new life. The cons include the possibility that the patient will be exposed to additional traumatic events in the context of CBT, which might exacerbate their symptoms. In these cases, therapists should empower their patient to make a decision that feels right for them based on the context in which they live and the other stressors in their life.

Modifications for Working in the Community

In some cases, there is a need to offer modifications to CBT when working in the community. When patients do not have a private space for doing their homework, the therapist might offer the patient to complete the homework in the clinic where possible. For instance, the therapist might arrange for a quiet space for the patient to sit and listen to their imaginal exposure homework. It might also help for the therapist to offer a computer for the patient to use for relevant *in vivo* exposure homework that requires internet connectivity. If a patient does not have a recorder, the therapist might consider lending the patient an audio recorder so that they can both record their imaginal exposure scripts and the patient can listen to them at home. These minimal modifications can go a long way toward building rapport and helping a patient feel cared for while completing emotionally difficult therapy.

Managing Other Clinicians Who Interface With the Patient

In many community mental health settings, the patient will see more than one member of a care team, including a psychiatrist, a case manager, a therapist, and possibly a nurse practitioner. When proceeding with CBT for PTSD, some members of the care team might have strong opinions about processing the trauma. For instance, one of my patients had a social worker who expressed some reservations about the patient doing imaginal exposure about her trauma. The social worker was not sure that the patient was emotionally ready to engage in this work. When the social worker brought this up to the patient, the patient also started to question her readiness to do this work and ultimately decided not to proceed with CBT. The patient might have been making the right decision for herself at that moment, but it is also possible that she might have benefited from the opportunity to safely share the story of what happened to her and to allow herself to heal.

In team-based approaches toward caring for PTSD, it can be helpful to maximize the support of other professionals to reinforce the patient's effective completion of therapy. With the patient's permission, it can be helpful to let the other team members know the types of exposures that the patient has been practicing so that the whole team can provide cheerleading and encouragement. Some members of the team might be able to provide logistical support to the patient, such as helping the patient to secure transportation to locations for *in vivo* exposures. It can also be helpful to work with a medication prescriber on establishing best practices for when a patient decides to take their medication in relation to when they do their CBT homework or come to sessions. The more that the team can rally around a common goal for the patient, the more empowered the patient will feel on their journey toward healing.

Balancing When to Be Flexible Versus Sticking to the Protocol

In community mental health consultations, I hear a lot of questions about when and whether it is appropriate to deviate from a CBT protocol. Examples of such considerations are given in Table 10.

Table 10. Considerations of deviation from the protocol for CBT for PTSD in community mental health

Type of deviation	Rationale for deviation	Rationale against deviation/ alternative solution
Not recording the session due to lack of technology	The patient is doing telehealth and does not have a recording device other than the one from which they are connecting (usually their phone).	The patient may benefit less from sessions if they cannot listen to the session content for homework; explore options for the clinic to provide the patient with a handheld audio recorder to borrow; explore whether the patient has any old/unused technology that still has a recording function.
Not recording the session due to anxiety	The patient is anxious that other people will gain access to the recording.	If recording on phone/tablet, make sure that the device is password protected.
Delaying the start of imaginal exposure	The patient is too anxious to begin imaginal exposure, or the therapist feels that the patient is not ready.	Delaying the start of imaginal exposure might increase anxiety about the procedure and result in increased dropout; it also conveys to the patient that the therapist is not sure whether the patient is ready for it, which reduces the patient's confidence.
Not doing imaginal exposures at all, and instead exclusively doing *in vivo* exposures/ behavioral activation	The therapist worries that the imaginal exposure will be too difficult for the patient.	By not trying imaginal exposures, the patient does not have the opportunity to potentially benefit from the healing opportunity of safely sharing their story.

continued on next page

Table 10. Continued

Type of deviation	Rationale for deviation	Rationale against deviation/ alternative solution
Frequent sessions focused on supportive psychotherapy as opposed to CBT	The patient might have frequent psychosocial stressors that warrant discussion and that might not fit within the CBT protocol.	If the patient has numerous off-protocol sessions, then they might not be considered to have actually received the CBT protocol and have no idea whether CBT alone would be effective for them; by focusing on problems unrelated to PTSD each week, there is less opportunity to directly target PTSD symptoms, which might reduce the impact of psychosocial stressors in the future.
Not prescribing homework	The therapist might feel that the patient does not have time to do CBT homework and therefore never prescribes it; alternatively, the therapist may stop prescribing homework if the patient is not doing it.	Doing homework in CBT for PTSD, especially imaginal exposure homework, reduces PTSD symptoms. If the therapist does not prescribe homework, or fails to check in on how the homework is going, the patient will potentially benefit less from the treatment. Instead of abandoning homework when it's not completed, brainstorm how the next session's homework can be made more realistic.

There are a few notable patterns reflected in these examples of considerations for deviation. First, a common reason why therapists are tempted to want to deviate from the CBT for PTSD protocol is the patient's anxiety (or the therapist's perceptions that patients may be anxious) about sticking to the prescribed protocol. Remember that avoiding something because it makes a patient anxious might increase their anxiety in the long run. Second, notice that many of these deviations tend to make the protocol less difficult or to reduce the workload for the patient and/or the therapist. CBT for PTSD involves more effort than other types of psychotherapy where there is no preparation for the session and no homework. While it might feel more comforting or easier to use a different approach in the short run, the cost of the easier path is that the patient has less opportunity to experience symptom resolution. An occasional off-protocol session is completely acceptable and appropriate in some circumstances (e.g., following the death of a loved one, the breakup of an important relationship, or significant job loss). However, when sessions become dominated by off-protocol procedures, the patient is no longer receiving CBT for PTSD. Third, I observe the same hesitation around imaginal exposures in private practice as I do in community mental health. Most therapists and patients are intimidated by imaginal exposures. That intimidation is exacerbated when the patient has numerous psychosocial stressors, which make the therapist worry about them. Rather than assuming that a patient is incapable of doing imaginal exposures, it can be more helpful to assume that if the procedure is too difficult or unhelpful, the patient and therapist will come up with an alternative plan.

Despite all the reasons listed here supporting decisions to stick to the evidence-based CBT protocol wherever possible, there are plenty of ways to be flexible in CBT for PTSD without limiting the effect of the treatment. If the patient initially struggles with imaginal exposures, you can consider a few alternative methods that stick to the spirit of approaching the memory but that might be less aversive:

- Instruct the patient to retell their story with their eyes open and using the past tense.
- Have the patient tell their story in a question-and-answer format, where the therapist asks a question and the patient provides the answer to continue the narrative.
- Have the patient write down their story.
- Have the patient draw their story.

Each of these procedures can be accomplished with a long-term goal of supporting the patient in working up to sharing their full imaginal exposure as written in the protocol.

Likewise, for a patient who is struggling with adherence to their *in vivo* homework, it might help them if you join them on an *in vivo* exposure. Alternatively, the patient might benefit from brainstorming around enlisting support from their own network of friends or family. It might also help them if you have a planned check-in phone call between sessions to ensure that the patient has completed the agreed-upon assignment.

The most important message around sticking to the protocol versus allowing flexibility is that there is a problem with both being too rigid and too flexible. Therapists who are too rigid will have patients who are intimidated to speak up and voice concerns, and their patients may be more likely to drop out of CBT for PTSD. Therapists who are too flexible will risk never actually administering CBT for PTSD. Like all good therapy, CBT for PTSD in the community requires ongoing assessment of the therapist's tendency toward rigidity and flexibility and helping the therapist to find a good middle ground that prioritizes the patient's needs.

Summary

There are more similarities than differences when working in community mental health and private practice in terms of the approach toward treating PTSD; however, PTSD is more prevalent in community mental health, which means that it constitutes a higher percentage of therapists' caseloads. In this chapter, I discussed the importance of trying to attend to patients' basic needs before they begin CBT for PTSD, such as having access to sufficient food and shelter. I also discussed the need to consider other members of the treatment team and that the therapist might need to work collaboratively with these to promote good outcomes for patients. I discussed some of the common examples of requests for deviation from the CBT for PTSD protocol that I receive in community health, as well as considerations about when to prioritize flexibility over sticking to the protocol.

15 Family Member Involvement in CBT for PTSD

PTSD affects the entire family system. As described in Chapter 1, a core symptom of PTSD includes difficulty with relating to other people. A second core symptom includes changes in cognitions about other people, including family. Thus, when providing CBT for PTSD, it is essential to consider the patient in the context of the larger family system.

Assessment Considerations

Family members can provide insight into symptoms of PTSD that a patient might not recognize. By involving family members to share their observations, the CBT therapist might gain insight into the complex impact of PTSD for the patient. Most of my assessments for adults with PTSD exclusively involve the patient, and I typically do not meet with family members until I understand a bit about the patient's unique experiences and the patient understands the treatment plan. While I do not include family members in assessment as the default, there are some situations in which it can be helpful.

First, if the patient with PTSD wants the therapist to hear from their family members about assessment-related considerations, this should always be honored. However, for adult patients with PTSD, the CBT therapist should typically meet individually with the patient first (if the patient is willing to do so) so as not to undermine the independence of the patient and to start the process of promoting empowerment in the patient. Then, the CBT therapist should inquire about why the patient feels that it is essential for the family members to weigh in on their observations and why the patient feels unsure about their ability to adequately explain aspects of their story. After meeting individually with the patient, the CBT therapist might then invite the family to share their perspectives and concerns.

The second situation in which it might be helpful to involve family members in the assessment is when the patient with PTSD reports fears about treatment provoking angry reactions. Some survivors with PTSD endorse trauma-related cognitions about being "out of control," or even "dangerous to others." In these cases, patients are sometimes worried about whether the treatment itself will exacerbate their symptoms and cause them to lash out in anger at loved ones. The CBT therapist should assess the most recent instance in which the patient engaged in angry behavior or behavior that they interpreted as evidence of having lost control. Many patients will not report examples consistent with their fears, but their fears persist nonetheless. Commonly, these patients will report intense avoidance of conflict because of their fears that conflict will result in them harming others. The patient might report beliefs such as, "If I don't get out of this situation, I'm going to lose it!" and might need to learn about their ability to tolerate negative emotions in important situations, as well as to learn that they are indeed in control of their behavior. However, if a patient reports having engaged in violent behaviors, it might be helpful or even essential to discuss safety with the adult family members or other necessary parties (for instance, child protective services) prior to proceeding with therapy from any modality. Chapter 11 discusses treatment of PTSD for survivors of intimate partner violence and includes some information that might be relevant to assessment in the family.

Psychoeducation Considerations

When patients want family members involved in treatment, the most helpful first step is to invite them for a psychoeducation session. Typically, this session occurs after the initial assessment and session 1. At this point in treatment, the CBT therapist has a general understanding of the patient's symptom profile and story, and the patient has a general understanding of the goals of treatment and the overall treatment plan. Prior to the family session, I typically coach the patient on what to expect in the family session.

I usually encourage the patient to take the lead in the family session. Ideally, the patient will have an opportunity to provide psychoeducation in their own words about *what* they are planning to do in treatment and *why* that plan will be implemented. There are two main reasons why this approach can be helpful. First, it ensures that the patient understands the psychoeducation sufficiently to explain it to another person. Second, since the patient is leading the conversation, they remain in control of what information is shared with their family (or not). When prepping the patient for this family meeting, I usually ask what they do and do not feel comfortable having their family member know about the trauma or the treatment. For instance, a patient might be willing to have their family member know that they were raped but might prefer not to disclose the identity of the rapist or the details surrounding the rape. The CBT therapist can coach the patient to redirect the conversation back to the goals of the session if the conversation veers in a direction that the patient prefers to keep private.

In terms of the content of psychoeducation, patients might find it helpful to share a bit of what they have learned about how avoidance and trauma-related cognitions maintain PTSD symptoms over time. They might also find it helpful to share that exposure practices and cognitive strategies can help in recovery from PTSD. The patient might desire to share some of what they have learned in terms of how exposure works and how the family member might be able to help them in this process (see more on this later in this chapter). In addition, it might be helpful to discuss the general approach to reducing avoidance of negative emotions as a core goal of CBT for PTSD. The patient might invite feedback from the family member about the potential impact of the treatment on the family member and take time to answer questions. If the patient or family member gets stuck in this conversation, the CBT therapist can step in as needed to provide clarification or to offer a reframing of content to promote mutual understanding.

In Vivo Exposure Considerations

Family members can be both a help and a hindrance for *in vivo* exposure practice depending on the patient's progress in treatment and unique relationship factors. In the early stages of *in vivo* exposures, having a family member join the patient can help with accountability and following through on the assignment. In later stages of *in vivo* exposures, the patient should be coached to practice weaning off of bringing a support person along for practice assignments to avoid the risk of the support person becoming a safety signal. In other words, the CBT therapist should coach the patient to work their way up to independence in exposure practices so that the patient can build confidence about their ability to survive and thrive if they encounter these situations alone in the future. Conducting independent *in vivo* exposures also reduces distraction and promotes opportunities for new learning, which is the core goal of these assignments.

Some family members have difficulty witnessing patients with PTSD as they struggle with difficult emotions in the context of *in vivo* exposures (or imaginal or interoceptive exposures). Those family members might default to a pattern of behavior that involves giving the patient with PTSD permission to avoid sources of distress. Usually, this tendency comes from a place of love and care, but it can backfire, making it harder for patients with PTSD to follow through on the objectives of CBT for PTSD. Especially if a patient with PTSD is tempted to skip an exposure practice, the temptation to push off the activity may feel impossible to overcome if a family member invites an opportunity for avoidance.

When a patient reveals that the dynamic with their family is enabling avoidance, I usually start with discussing this pattern with the patient. I normalize that this is an extremely common dynamic in families with people who love each other, even if it is not ultimately helpful. Then, I ask the patient to identify their objectives, given that the family dynamic is making it harder for them to complete *in vivo* exposure practice.

Some patients share this dynamic with me because they want me to support them in their decision to drop out of treatment or to continue in a treatment that does not involve exposure practice. It might be easier for them to tell me that their parent or spouse does not want them to do *in vivo* exposures than it is for them to voice this as their own concern. In those situations, I remind the patient that they are in control of the therapy and that if they choose to stop the therapy, I will fully support them in that decision, but that I hope that we can find a way to collaborate in a treatment plan to move forward. I also remind them that I will never force them (or even pressure them) to engage in an exposure that they are not ready to complete.

Other patients recognize that they need to continue doing exposures and must find a way to communicate the importance of these practices to their families. In these cases, we can spend time on assertive communication training. This might involve teaching patients the DEAR MAN skill from dialectical behavior therapy for making an assertive request (Linehan, 1993). We might also need to do role play practice to help the patient in finding an assertive voice that works for them. Finally, we might need to make a coping card with a helpful reminder to them to use when a family member encourages them to avoid treatment. For instance, "If I'm going to get better, I need to practice facing my fears."

Still other patients find that the backlash that they get to doing *in vivo* exposures is part of a long-standing family dynamic that is challenging to address in individual therapy. *In vivo* exposures might place a burden on the family in terms of time away from the family, borrowing a family vehicle, or using family resources that might be scarce. In these instances, the CBT therapist might help the patient to brainstorm how recovery from PTSD might ultimately improve family functioning. The patient might find it beneficial to share their vision with their family about how making changes now may require some sacrifices in the short run, but that the goal of the treatment is to help everyone in the family thrive. If the patient has concrete examples of how they envision recovery from PTSD will improve their ability to contribute to the family, it can be helpful for them to consider sharing that vision with the family to improve buy-in. The patient might also reckon with the reality that their family members also have life complications that might make it such that they cannot prioritize being supportive of the patient even if they might wish to make this their priority.

If a patient finds it helpful to have another psychoeducation session with the family to reset expectations around *in vivo* exposures, this can help get treatment back on track. The goals for this session might include providing more details about why and how we conduct *in vivo* exposures. We might also include an opportunity in the family session for the patient to voice a request expressing how the family member can be most supportive of them in their *in vivo* practice.

Imaginal Exposure Considerations

As briefly mentioned in Chapter 1, the impact of traumas can be so intense that they can leave survivors feeling very isolated. As part of the healing process, some patients with PTSD have a strong desire to share the details of what they experienced with loved ones. It might seem natural to even consider allowing family members to listen to the audio recording of the imaginal exposure. Generally, I tend to actively discourage this practice for a few core reasons:

- Family members are not trained mental health professionals and might not know what to say or do when learning of the imaginal exposure, even if they want to be helpful.
- In an attempt to be helpful, family members might default to cliché remarks that could inadvertently be harmful to the patient (i.e., "Everything happens for a reason"; "If you keep thinking positively, things will get better soon," etc.).
- Family members could become extremely emotionally dysregulated after learning about horrible events happening to the patient. Given that they are unable to provide care to the family members due to dual-relationship ethical issues, except in extraordinary circumstances when other therapists are unavailable, the therapist should be thoughtful about the emotional toll of detailed disclosure about the trauma on the patient's family.
- Unlike the therapist and the patient, the family member will be unlikely to repeatedly engage with the memory of the trauma, which means that the distress that is caused for them by a one-time session is unlikely to resolve.

When a patient expresses a desire to share their imaginal exposure recording with a family member, I first want to understand why they are tempted to do so. In some cases, patients want to share the recording because they feel overwhelmed by the practice and desire support from a family member. In those cases, we can brainstorm ways to request support from the family or other people without having to share the graphic details of the trauma. In other cases, it feels important to the patient that someone else genuinely understands their experience. In this case, it can be helpful to understand how the patient perceives that this would help them. Perhaps the patient feels that if their family understood the severity of what they survived, it would lighten the load that the patient carries. In this case, it might be helpful to have a discussion with the patient to explore the likelihood of that outcome, which is possible but not definitive.

Thus, instead of the patient sharing the actual audio recording of the imaginal exposure, I ask my patients about what they hope sharing the recording will accomplish. In Chapter 5, I discussed how *in vivo* exposures that involve communications with other people can be complicated if the patient has a subtle goal of hoping to elicit a particular reaction from other people. I mentioned that when a patient has an *in vivo* exposure around communication, the goal should be geared toward the communication itself (e.g., "I can handle talking about this with other people"; "I am able to make an assertive request," etc.), as opposed to the outcome of the communication. When it comes to an instinct to share an imaginal exposure script, it might be helpful to encourage the patient to consider whether there are less intense ways of communicating their important message rather than a detailed play-by-play of the worst event that ever happened to them.

Behavioral Activation Considerations (Including Use of Rewards)

As mentioned in Chapter 8, behavioral activation can be a helpful strategy for combating comorbid depression symptoms and for increasing self-esteem. While the principles of behavioral activation are simple, following through on commitments to complete agreed-upon activities can present challenges when patients are struggling with comorbid depression symptoms. Family members can offer several sources of support to patients with PTSD as they complete behavioral activation activities.

First, family members can offer a source of public accountability. When a patient with PTSD tells their family member that they are planning to complete an activity, this disclosure alone might increase the likelihood of following through. This can be an especially effective intervention if the patient suspects that their family member will check-in with them about whether they did the activity and how it went. The patient should negotiate with their family member for the appropriate level of support, and the CBT therapist can help navigate this conversation if desired by the patient. Some patients will find it helpful for their family members to directly ask them about whether the behavioral activation assignment was completed. Other patients may be reluctant to have someone else "police" their behavior and prefer to simply share what they are planning without an expectation that the family member will check in with them. Either of these options can be helpful to patients and family members alike, if both agree to the expectations in advance and each has permission to communicate with the other party when the arrangement is not working as desired.

Second, family members can help patients with PTSD to select activities for behavioral activation that are realistic and tied to the patients' larger system of goals and values. Family members have a wealth of historical knowledge about activities that patients previously engaged in and found enjoyable or that contributed positively to self-esteem. Thus, when a patient aspires to complete behavioral activation assignments but is stuck in terms of which activities to select, family members might offer helpful suggestions. Family members also have a global sense of the rest of the patient's life in a way that a CBT therapist (who has a targeted focus on treating PTSD symptoms) might not. As such, family members can weigh in on which activities seem feasible for the patient in the context of their larger life commitments and which ones might be better suited for the future.

Third, family members can join in the activity to increase the patient's enjoyment and pleasure. While some activities might be most enjoyable when completed independently, other activities are amplified when conducted in partnership with a trusted person. Due to trauma-related cognitions, patients with PTSD might be reluctant to ask for help and might avoid being a burden on other people. The CBT therapist can support the patient, with their permission, by coaching the patient to invite family members for behavioral activation activities even when these trauma-related cognitions make it challenging. In some cases, it might even help to have the patient "blame" the therapist for needing to make the request initially. Whereas I eventually hope that the patient will learn the skill of assertive requests without the need to caveat the requests as having come from an external source, blaming the therapist for the request might allow the patient to practice making assertive requests in a manner that feels less threatening to them initially. For instance, if the patient's request is rejected, it might not feel as negative if they perceive that it was not their idea in the first place.

Fourth, family members can help patients with PTSD to reward themselves when they accomplish the goals of behavioral activation. For most people, self-reward comes as an extreme challenge. Sometimes families provide subtle and overt messages about rewards being childish or self-indulgent. In such instances, the CBT therapist might help the patient by communicating to them and their family about the necessity of rewarding positive behaviors if someone hopes to continue those behaviors in the future. The family members might also have insights into types of rewards that would be effective for the patient.

Extinction Bursts in Family Members

When one member of a family starts to change their behavior, it can upset the homeostasis in the family unit. Family members might have adopted certain patterns in their behavior to accommodate patients with PTSD and might observe that things feel less comfortable to everyone as the patient makes new changes in their behavior. The patient and their family members might have complicated feelings about those changes. On the one hand, a family member might feel relieved that the patient is finally getting the necessary help to promote healing and restoration. On the other hand, the patient might experience a newfound empowerment and independence that is unusual in the family and may increase anxiety.

Changes to the typical family dynamic might cause an extinction burst in the family. An extinction burst is a sudden increase in behavior that occurs when the rules of engagement change, and when behaviors that used to result in one outcome are no longer associated with that outcome. For instance, when a family member asks a patient with PTSD to do something and the patient with PTSD immediately complies, even though they do not want to complete the request, this results in an expectation in the family member that the patient will agree to their requests in the future as well. If a patient with PTSD is practicing finding their voice and asserting themselves, a family member might be shocked and disappointed if the patient does not comply as is typical. Because the family member is surprised, they might escalate their behavior (an extinction burst) and yell at the patient or increase the intensity of their request. This can be upsetting for both the patient and the family member.

There are numerous disruptions to the family dynamic that can be healthy in the long run but that require some adjustments in the short run. For instance, some romantic partners might feel threatened that the patient will no longer be interested in continuing in the relationship, as they are now feeling more confident. Those partners might worry that the patient no longer "needs them." Whereas the patient might not need them in the same manner as before treatment, the patient may still hope to stay in the relationship and cultivate a new, healthier dynamic. Other partners might feel frustrated that the patient is engaging in more assertive behavior as opposed to "going with the flow." These partners might feel rejected by the patient who had traditionally been very accommodating to their requests. Improved confidence might result in changes in intimate moments or in confidence to wear certain clothes that might be surprising to patients' partners. These are just some of the examples of disruptions to a typical family dynamic that might require a family session (or family therapy, separate from individual therapy with the patient, ideally with another therapist) to help the family process.

Some of the changes that emerge for patients and their families during or following CBT for PTSD are best addressed in family therapy, whereas others might be addressed well in a single psychoeducation session. The patient and their family should be given information about the differences between a psychoeducation session, wherein the therapist is ultimately aligned with the patient and serving as an advocate for the patient, and family therapy, where the therapist is representing the stakes of the family as a whole and not biased by the perspective of any one family member. For some families, a psychoeducation session can accomplish a few core goals:

- Normalizing the idea that when one member of a family gets treatment, it often results in both positive and negative consequences for the family
- Provision of reassurance that, after an adjustment period, the family tends to find a new normal that is healthier in the long run
- Giving information about how, if they notice that the new normal is especially painful or if they are having significant difficulty with adjusting or handling family matters for another reason, couples or family therapy can be a great option for them. The therapist should ideally provide some referrals to the family proactively, as opposed to waiting for them to ask. It might also be important to remind the family that sometimes waiting lists for family or couples therapy can be long, and it might be better to get on a waiting list sooner rather than later. Families might also benefit from knowing that a common issue with family therapy is that families wait until it is too late to start and things have occurred that are so hurtful that it is very difficult to recover.

Summary

In this chapter, I discussed the significant impact of PTSD on the entire family unit. I reviewed considerations for involvement of family members in assessment and briefly outlined the practicalities of their inclusion to promote independence in the patient. Then I discussed a psychoeducation session with the family, which is the most common way that family members are involved in CBT for PTSD. I detailed how family members can support patients with PTSD as they implement *in vivo* exposures, imaginal exposures, and behavioral activation. Finally, I explored how it can upset the entire family system when a patient with PTSD gets the treatment that they need and the family might benefit from an opportunity to process this in a psychoeducation session or in family therapy. Involvement of family members can be essential for the optimal treatment of some patients with PTSD, and they can be a source of support to patients that is priceless when they are thoughtfully coached to give it.

16 Self-Care in Working With Trauma Survivors Using CBT for PTSD

Therapists must practice good self-care to stay focused on their patients' needs. When therapists hear horrifying stories about traumatic experiences, it becomes essential for them to find a way to invest in their own mental health. In this chapter, I review some key considerations for promoting self-care while providing CBT for PTSD.

A Personal Anecdote

I remember a patient whom I was seeing while I was a predoctoral intern. She was receiving treatment for symptoms of borderline personality disorder and had a significant history of trauma, including trauma perpetrated by a current partner. The PTSD symptoms that she struggled with were exacerbated every day by her partner as he continued to engage in abusive behavior toward her. The patient presented in a very timid manner and was always extremely polite and respectful, but she became filled with fear as we discussed the application of some CBT skills to her home life. It became clear that it was not safe for her to be assertive in this relationship, and she was not ready to leave the relationship. She felt trapped, and as a result, I felt trapped too.

After one of our sessions, I took a long drive to my parents' house to visit them for the weekend. I was traveling solo, and I could not stop thinking about this patient. I realized that I was very scared for her safety, but I felt that there was nothing I could do to help her. I remember thinking that this patient had experienced so many unfair situations – it filled me with rage and extreme sadness. I started sobbing on the drive and had to use slow breathing to compose myself. I realized that I needed to figure out a way to give myself permission to feel whatever I needed to feel, but also that I needed to make sure that I was taking care of myself.

One of the most freeing realizations that I had from working with this patient was the following: This patient's PTSD symptoms were contributing to her decision to remain in an abusive relationship. If I could find a way to become an expert in treating PTSD, I would always have an option to help patients with their PTSD. For this patient, the fact that we were *not* providing CBT for PTSD (for various legitimate reasons related to the patient's self-reported readiness for such treatment, among other factors) was part of what was contributing to my sense of helplessness for her.

As therapists, we will always have patients who affect us deeply, which is not an indication that we are doing something wrong. However, if you know that stories of trauma are difficult to hear (as they are for most of us), then the best way to work through this is to use the treatments that have the strongest evidence base for PTSD. When we know that we are providing the best possible treatment for a deeply painful condition, it builds confidence in holding the pain with our patients.

Some Important Reminders About Self-Care When Working With Patients With PTSD

The first time that you hear the details of a trauma might be difficult. As you sit with the patient in the revisiting process, wherein they tell the details of their experience repeatedly, it typically becomes easier. The reason for this is twofold: (1) the patient is starting to experience some symptom relief; and (2) the therapist starts to react less to a horrible story as they hear it repeatedly. At the Center for the Treatment and Study of Anxiety, we always remind therapists to trust the process and that when they allow themselves to follow the protocol, the patient gets better. This builds the therapist's confidence as well. Some therapists have reported that you might not believe in the benefit of CBT for PTSD until you have witnessed it firsthand in your patient. In this manner, the best possible self-care when working with patients with PTSD is to give them the highest-quality therapy that has the greatest likelihood of improving symptoms quickly (namely, CBT).

Personal Limits as Self-Care

It is important for us all to have our own limits around what does and does not work for us when providing CBT for PTSD. It might be challenging for you to work with certain trauma types if you are going through a difficult period in your own life. For instance, if a therapist recently experienced a miscarriage, it might be difficult to help a patient process the trauma of a miscarriage. Likewise, a therapist who has experienced being mugged might not feel emotionally ready to help a patient who is sorting through their PTSD while the therapist is still healing. Therapists must be allowed to set their own limits about what is possible for them and to allow those limits to change as needed.

I hope that most therapists reading this book have already developed a form of self-care that is suitable to their needs. However, sometimes therapists, like the rest of the population, fall into a rut of self-care where things that used to work for them are no longer helpful. If you have noticed that you need more proactive opportunities to promote self-care, you might consider following the behavioral activation guidelines that I outlined in Chapter 8. The key to self-care is finding something that is effective for you and that you feel comfortable with and able to continue using in the future.

Consultation as Self-Care

One form of self-care that can be extremely helpful for therapists is to get consultation on their cases. This can take the form of a therapist process group, group supervision, or individual case consultations. Given that we are ethically and legally required to maintain confidentiality, it can be extremely helpful to have a professional consultation service to ensure that you are making thoughtful decisions when delivering CBT for PTSD.

Therapy for Self-Care

It can be challenging for therapists to admit that they need professional support when they are used to serving in a helping role. Whereas some therapists are mandated to receive therapy as part of their professional training, this is not a requirement in most programs. Especially when therapists notice that the content of therapy affects their ability to provide therapy, it is important to consider getting professional support. This is no more likely to emerge in the context of CBT for PTSD than in other types of treatment for PTSD, but it might be more likely when working with PTSD in general.

Summary

When working with PTSD, it is essential for the therapist to attend to self-care. The best kind of self-care is to deliver effective treatment for PTSD and to witness the psychological healing that follows in the patient. While delivering CBT for PTSD, it is essential for therapists to attend to their own limits and needs, including getting consultation and support from other professions. That support can also take the form of receiving formal therapy when desired and/or needed by the therapist.

References

Adams, R. E., & Boscarino, J. A. (2006). Predictors of PTSD and delayed PTSD after disaster: The impact of exposure and psychosocial resources. *Journal of Nervous and Mental Disease, 194*(7), 485. https://doi.org/10.1097/01.nmd.0000228503.95503.e9

Almeida, J., Barber, C., Rosen, R. K., Nicolopoulos, A., & O'Brien, K. H. M. (2023). "In the moment I wanted to kill myself, and then after I didn't": A qualitative investigation of suicide planning, method choice, and method substitution among adolescents hospitalized following a suicide attempt. *Youth & Society, 55*(1), 29–43. https://doi.org/10.1177/0044118X211035950

American Psychiatric Association. (2013). *Diagnostic and statistical manual of mental disorders* (5th ed.) [DSM-5]. https://doi.org/10.1176/appi.books.9780890425596

American Psychiatric Association. (2022). *Diagnostic and statistical manual of mental disorders* (5th ed., text rev.) [DSM-5-TR]. https://doi.org/10.1176/appi.books.9780890425787

American Psychological Association. (2017). *Clinical practice guideline for the treatment of posttraumatic stress disorder (PTSD).* https://www.apa.org/ptsd-guideline/ptsd.pdf

Badour, C. L., Blonigen, D. M., Boden, M. T., Feldner, M. T., & Bonn-Miller, M. O. (2012). A longitudinal test of the bi-directional relations between avoidance coping and PTSD severity during and after PTSD treatment. *Behaviour Research and Therapy, 50*(10), 610–616. https://doi.org/10.1016/j.brat.2012.06.006

Ballentine, E., Feler, B., Narine, K., & Brown, L. A. (2025). A qualitative study of ecological momentary assessment of suicide risk for persons living with HIV in Philadelphia, PA, USA: Feasibility, acceptability, and ethical implications. *Journal of the Association of Nurses in AIDS Care*. Advance online publication. https://doi.org/10.1097/JNC.0000000000000586

Bargai, N., Ben-Shakhar, G., & Shalev, A. Y. (2007). Posttraumatic stress disorder and depression in battered women: The mediating role of learned helplessness. *Journal of Family Violence, 22*(5), 267–275. https://doi.org/10.1007/s10896-007-9078-y

Barlow, D. H., Farchione, T. J., Sauer-Zavala, S., Latin, H. M., Ellard, K. K., Bullis, J. R., Bentley, K. H., Boettcher, H. T., & Cassiello-Robbins, C. (2017). Module 5: Countering emotional behaviors: (Corresponds to chapter 9 of the UP workbook). In D. H. Barlow, T. J. Farchione, S. Sauer-Zavala, H. Murray Latin, K. K. Ellard, J. R. Bullis, K. H. Bentley, H. T. Boettcher, C. Cassiello-Robbins, D. H. Barlow, T. J. Farchione, S. Sauer-Zavala, H. M. Latin, K. K. Ellard, J. R. Bullis, K. H. Bentley, H. T. Boettcher, & C. Cassiello-Robbins (Eds.), *Unified protocol for transdiagnostic treatment of emotional disorders: Therapist guide* (2nd ed., pp. 113–130). Oxford University Press. https://doi.org/10.1093/med-psych/9780190685973.003.0010

Barlow, D. H., Sauer-Zavala, S., Farchione, T. J., Latin, H. M., Ellard, K. K., Bullis, J. R., Bentley, K. H., Boettcher, H. T., & Cassiello-Robbins, C. (2017). Putting it into practice—Emotion exposures. In D. H. Barlow, T. J. Farchione, S. Sauer-Zavala, H. Murray Latin, K. K. Ellard, J. R. Bullis, K. H. Bentley, H. T. Boettcher, & C. Cassiello-Robbins (Eds.),

Unified protocol for transdiagnostic treatment of emotional disorders: Workbook (2nd ed. pp. 125–136). Oxford University Press. https://doi.org/10.1093/med-psych/9780190686017.003.0011

Basile, K. C., Smith, S. G., Kresnow, M., Khatiwada, S., & Leemis, R. W. (2022). *The National Intimate Partner and Sexual Violence Survey: 2016/2017 report on sexual violence.* National Center for Injury Prevention and Control, Centers for Disease Control and Prevention. https://stacks.cdc.gov/view/cdc/124625

Bates, E. A. (2016). Current controversies within intimate partner violence: Overlooking bidirectional violence. *Journal of Family Violence, 31*(8), 937–940. https://doi.org/10.1007/s10896-016-9862-7

Beck, A. T., & Steer, R. A. (1991). *Beck Scale for Suicide Ideation manual.* Pearson.

Beck, J. G., Palyo, S. A., Canna, M. A., Blanchard, E. B., & Gudmundsdottir, B. (2006). What factors are associated with the maintenance of PTSD after a motor vehicle accident? The role of sex differences in a help-seeking population. *Journal of Behavior Therapy and Experimental Psychiatry, 37*(3), 256–266. https://doi.org/10.1016/j.jbtep.2005.04.001

Beck, J. S. (2010). Cognitive therapy. In *The Corsini encyclopedia of psychology* (pp. 1–3). Wiley. https://doi.org/10.1002/9780470479216.corpsy0198

Becker, C. B., Darius, E., & Schaumberg, K. (2007). An analog study of patient preferences for exposure versus alternative treatments for posttraumatic stress disorder. *Behaviour Research and Therapy, 45*(12), 2861–2873. https://doi.org/10.1016/j.brat.2007.05.006

Bender, T. W., Fitzpatrick, S., Hartmann, M.-A., Hames, J., Bodell, L., Selby, E. A., & Joiner, T. E. (2019). Does it hurt to ask? An analysis of iatrogenic risk during suicide risk assessment. *Neurology, Psychiatry and Brain Research, 33*, 73–81. https://doi.org/10.1016/j.npbr.2019.07.005

Benjet, C., Bromet, E., Karam, E. G., Kessler, R. C., McLaughlin, K. A., Ruscio, A. M., Shahly, V., Stein, D. J., Petukhova, M., Hill, E., Alonso, J., Atwoli, L., Bunting, B., Bruffaerts, R., Caldas-de-Almeida, J. M., de Girolamo, G., Florescu, S., Gureje, O., Huang, Y., … Koenen, K. C. (2016). The epidemiology of traumatic event exposure worldwide: Results from the World Mental Health Survey Consortium. *Psychological Medicine, 46*(2), 327–343. https://doi.org/10.1017/S0033291715001981

Betz, M. E., Stanley, I. H., Anestis, M. D., Bryan, C. J., Buck-Atkinson, J., Carey, N., Ghahramanlou-Holloway, M., Morrissey, B. H., Holloway, K., Houtsma, C., Kennedy, R., Paine, C. M., Ramchand, R., Simonetti, J., Walsh, A., & Wright-Kelly, E. (2023). Firearm suicide prevention in the U.S. military: Recommendations from a national summit. *Military Medicine, 188*(9–10), 231–235. https://doi.org/10.1093/milmed/usac371

Bilek, E. L., Tomlinson, R. C., Whiteman, A. S., Johnson, T. D., Benedict, C., Phan, K. L., Monk, C. S., & Fitzgerald, K. D. (2022). Exposure-focused CBT outperforms relaxation-based control in an RCT of treatment for child and adolescent anxiety. *Journal of Clinical Child and Adolescent Psychology: The Official Journal for the Society of Clinical Child and Adolescent Psychology, American Psychological Association, Division 53, 51*(4), 410–418. https://doi.org/10.1080/15374416.2021.1901230

Bluett, E. J., Zoellner, L. A., & Feeny, N. C. (2014). Does change in distress matter? Mechanisms of change in prolonged exposure for PTSD. *Journal of Behavior Therapy and Experimental Psychiatry, 45*(1), https://doi.org/10.1016/j.jbtep.2013.09.003

Bonde, J. P. E., Jensen, J. H., Smid, G. E., Flachs, E. M., Elklit, A., Mors, O., & Videbech, P. (2022). Time course of symptoms in posttraumatic stress disorder with delayed expression: A systematic review. *Acta Psychiatrica Scandinavica, 145*(2), 116–131. https://doi.org/10.1111/acps.13372

Bouton, M. E. (1988). Context and ambiguity in the extinction of emotional learning: Implications for exposure therapy. *Behaviour Research and Therapy, 26*(2), 137–149. https://doi.org/10.1016/0005-7967(88)90113-1

Bovin, M. J., Marx, B. P., Weathers, F. W., Gallagher, M. W., Rodriguez, P., Schnurr, P. P., & Keane, T. M. (2016). Psychometric properties of the PTSD checklist for Diagnostic and statistical manual of mental disorders – Fifth edition (PCL-5) in veterans. *Psychological Assessment, 28*(11), 1379–1391. https://doi.org/10.1037/pas0000254

Brave Heart, M. Y. H., & DeBruyn, L. (1998). The American Indian holocaust: Healing historical unresolved grief. *American Indian and Alaska Native Mental Health Research, 8*(2), 60–82. https://doi.org/10.5820/aian.0802.1998.60

Bredemeier, K., & Miller, I. W. (2015). Executive function and suicidality: A systematic qualitative review. *Clinical Psychology Review, 40*, 170–183. https://doi.org/10.1016/j.cpr.2015.06.005

Brewerton, T. D., Perlman, M. M., Gavidia, I., Suro, G., Genet, J., & Bunnell, D. W. (2020). The association of traumatic events and posttraumatic stress disorder with greater eating disorder and comorbid symptom severity in residential eating disorder treatment centers. *International Journal of Eating Disorders, 53*(12), 2061–2066. https://doi.org/10.1002/eat.23401

Briant, K. J., Halter, A., Marchello, N., Escareño, M., & Thompson, B. (2016). The power of digital storytelling as a culturally relevant health promotion tool. *Health Promotion Practice, 17*(6), 793–801. https://doi.org/10.1177/1524839916658023

Brown, L. A., Belli, G. M., Asnaani, A., & Foa, E. B. (2019). A review of the role of negative cognitions about oneself, others, and the world in the treatment of PTSD. *Cognitive Therapy and Research, 43*(1), 143–173. https://doi.org/10.1007/s10608-018-9938-1

Brown, L. A., Chen, S., Narine, K., Contractor, A. A., & Oslin, D. (2020). DSM-5 PTSD symptom clusters and suicidal ideation in veterans. *Psychiatry Research, 288*, 112942. https://doi.org/10.1016/j.psychres.2020.112942

Brown, L. A., Contractor, A., & Benhamou, K. (2018). Posttraumatic stress disorder clusters and suicidal ideation. *Psychiatry Research, 270*, 238–245. https://doi.org/10.1016/j.psychres.2018.09.030

Brown, L. A., Fernandez, C. A., Kohn, R., Saldivia, S., & Vicente, B. (2018). Pre-disaster PTSD as a moderator of the relationship between natural disaster and suicidal ideation over time. *Journal of Affective Disorders, 230*, 7–14. https://doi.org/10.1016/j.jad.2017.12.096

Brown, L. A., Jerud, A., Asnaani, A., Petersen, J., Zang, Y., & Foa, E. B. (2018). Changes in posttraumatic stress disorder (PTSD) and depressive symptoms over the course of prolonged exposure. *Journal of Consulting and Clinical Psychology, 86*(5), 452–463. https://doi.org/10.1037/ccp0000292

Brown, L. A., LeBeau, R., Liao, B., Niles, A. N., Glenn, D., & Craske, M. G. (2016). A comparison of the nature and correlates of panic attacks in the context of panic disorder and social anxiety disorder. *Psychiatry Research, 235*, 69–76. https://doi.org/10.1016/j.psychres.2015.11.048

Brown, L. A., Taylor, D. J., Bryan, C., Wiley, J. F., Pruiksma, K., Khazem, L., Baker, J. C., Young, J., & O'Leary, K. (2022). Digital phenotyping to improve prediction of suicidal urges in treatment: Study protocol. *Aggression and Violent Behavior, 66*, 101733. https://doi.org/10.1016/j.avb.2022.101733

Brown, L. A., Zhu, Y., Narine, K., Simon, S., & Akpoduado, E. (2022). Timing of suicidal ideation among persons living with HIV. *The Behavior Therapist, 45*(8), 298–306.

Bryan, C. J. (2019). A preliminary validation study of two ultra-brief measures of suicide risk: The Suicide and Perceived Burdensomeness Visual Analog Scales. *Suicide & Life-Threatening Behavior, 49*(2), 343–352. https://doi.org/10.1111/sltb.12447

Bryan, C. J., Butner, J. E., May, A. M., Rugo, K. F., Harris, J. A., Oakey, D. N., Rozek, D. C., & Bryan, A. O. (2020). Nonlinear change processes and the emergence of suicidal behavior: A conceptual model based on the fluid vulnerability theory of suicide. *New Ideas in Psychology, 57*, 100758. https://doi.org/10.1016/j.newideapsych.2019.100758

Bryan, C. J., Mintz, J., Clemans, T. A., Leeson, B., Burch, T. S., Williams, S. R., Maney, E., & Rudd, M. D. (2017). Effect of crisis response planning vs. contracts for safety on suicide risk in U.S. army soldiers: A randomized clinical trial. *Journal of Affective Disorders, 212*, 64–72. https://doi.org/10.1016/j.jad.2017.01.028

Bryant, R. A., & Harvey, A. G. (2003). The influence of litigation on maintenance of posttraumatic stress disorder. *Journal of Nervous and Mental Disease, 191*(3), 191. https://doi.org/10.1097/01.NMD.0000055080.96195.EE

Campbell, J. C., Webster, D. W., & Glass, N. (2009). The danger assessment: Validation of a lethality risk assessment instrument for intimate partner femicide. *Journal of Interpersonal Violence, 24*(4), 653–674. https://doi.org/10.1177/0886260508317180

Cattaneo, L., Bell, M., Goodman, L., & Dutton, M. (2007). Intimate partner violence victims' accuracy in assessing their risk of re-abuse. *Journal of Family Violence, 22*, 429–440. https://doi.org/10.1007/s10896-007-9097-8

Chioneso, N. A., Hunter, C. D., Gobin, R. L., McNeil Smith, S., Mendenhall, R., & Neville, H. A. (2020). Community healing and resistance through storytelling: A framework to address racial trauma in Africana communities. *Journal of Black Psychology, 46*(2–3), 95–121. https://doi.org/10.1177/0095798420929468

Clark, D. M., Layard, R., Smithies, R., Richards, D. A., Suckling, R., & Wright, B. (2009). Improving access to psychological therapy: Initial evaluation of two UK demonstration sites. *Behaviour Research and Therapy, 47*(11), 910–920. https://doi.org/10.1016/j.brat.2009.07.010

Coalition for National Trauma Research. (2024). Trauma statistics & facts. Coalition for National Trauma Research website. https://www.nattrauma.org/trauma-statistics-facts/

Cohen, J. A., Mannarino, A. P., & Deblinger, E. (2006). *Treating trauma and traumatic grief in children and adolescents*. 2nd ed. Guilford Press.

Cooper, A. A., Kline, A. C., Graham, B., Bedard-Gilligan, M., Mello, P. G., Feeny, N. C., & Zoellner, L. A. (2017). Homework "dose," type, and helpfulness as predictors of clinical outcomes in prolonged exposure for PTSD. *Behavior Therapy, 48*(2), 182–194. https://doi.org/10.1016/j.beth.2016.02.013

Craig, S. L., Austin, A., Levenson, J., Leung, V. W. Y., Eaton, A. D., & D'Souza, S. A. (2020). Frequencies and patterns of adverse childhood events in LGBTQ+ youth. *Child Abuse & Neglect, 107*, 104623. https://doi.org/10.1016/j.chiabu.2020.104623

Craske, M. G., Farchione, T. J., Allen, L. B., Barrios, V., Stoyanova, M., & Rose, R. (2007). Cognitive behavioral therapy for panic disorder and comorbidity: More of the same or less of more? *Behaviour Research and Therapy, 45*(6), 1095–1109. https://doi.org/10.1016/j.brat.2006.09.006

Cully, J. A., & Teten, A. L. (2008). *A therapist's guide to brief cognitive behavioral therapy*. Department of Veterans Affairs, South Central Mental Illness Research, Education, and Clinical Center.

Cusack, K., Jonas, D. E., Forneris, C. A., Wines, C., Sonis, J., Middleton, J. C., Feltner, C., Brownley, K. A., Olmsted, K. R., Greenblatt, A., Weil, A., & Gaynes, B. N. (2016).

Psychological treatments for adults with posttraumatic stress disorder: A systematic review and meta-analysis. *Clinical Psychology Review, 43*, 128–141. https://doi.org/10.1016/j.cpr.2015.10.003

Dazzi, T., Gribble, R., Wessely, S., & Fear, N. T. (2014). Does asking about suicide and related behaviours induce suicidal ideation? What is the evidence? *Psychological Medicine, 44*(16), 3361–3363. https://doi.org/10.1017/S0033291714001299

Deisenhammer, E. A., Kuen, D., Ing, C.-M., Kemmler, G., Defrancesco, M., von Gleissenthall, G., & Weiss, E. M. (2016). Stability in the choice of method during the period preceding a suicide attempt and in attempt repeaters. *European Journal of Psychiatry, 30*(3), 205–217.

de Kleine, R. A., Hendriks, L., Becker, E. S., Broekman, T. G., & van Minnen, A. (2017). Harm expectancy violation during exposure therapy for posttraumatic stress disorder. *Journal of Anxiety Disorders, 49*, 48–52. https://doi.org/10.1016/j.janxdis.2017.03.008

Departments of Veterans Affairs and Defense (VA/DoD). (2023). *VA/DoD clinical practice guideline for management of posttraumatic stress disorder and acute stress disorder*. https://www.ptsd.va.gov/professional/treat/txessentials/cpg_ptsd_management.asp

Dickie, E. W., Brunet, A., Akerib, V., & Armony, J. L. (2008). An fMRI investigation of memory encoding in PTSD: Influence of symptom severity. *Neuropsychologia, 46*(5), 1522–1531. https://doi.org/10.1016/j.neuropsychologia.2008.01.007

Difede, J., & Barocas, D. (1999). Acute intrusive and avoidant PTSD symptoms as predictors of chronic PTSD following burn injury. *Journal of Traumatic Stress, 12*(2), 363–369. https://doi.org/10.1023/A:1024788812393

Duek, O., Spiller, T. R., Pietrzak, R. H., Fried, E. I., & Harpaz-Rotem, I. (2021). Network analysis of PTSD and depressive symptoms in 158,139 treatment-seeking veterans with PTSD. *Depression and Anxiety, 38*(5), 554–562. https://doi.org/10.1002/da.23112

Dunmore, E., Clark, D. M., & Ehlers, A. (1999). Cognitive factors involved in the onset and maintenance of posttraumatic stress disorder (PTSD) after physical or sexual assault. *Behaviour Research and Therapy, 37*(9), 809–829. https://doi.org/10.1016/S0005-7967(98)00181-8

East, L., Jackson, D., O'Brien, L., & Peters, K. (2010). Storytelling: An approach that can help to develop resilience. *Nurse Researcher, 17*(3), 17–25. https://doi.org/10.7748/nr2010.04.17.3.17.c7742

Edmondson, D., & Känel, R. von. (2017). Post-traumatic stress disorder and cardiovascular disease. *The Lancet Psychiatry, 4*(4), 320–329. https://doi.org/10.1016/S2215-0366(16)30377-7

Ehlers, A., Clark, D. M., Hackmann, A., McManus, F., & Fennell, M. (2005). Cognitive therapy for post-traumatic stress disorder: Development and evaluation. *Behaviour Research and Therapy, 43*(4), 413–431. https://doi.org/10.1016/j.brat.2004.03.006

Ehring, T., Frank, S., & Ehlers, A. (2008). The role of rumination and reduced concreteness in the maintenance of posttraumatic stress disorder and depression following trauma. *Cognitive Therapy and Research, 32*(4), 488–506. https://doi.org/10.1007/s10608-006-9089-7

Elliott, J. E., Opel, R. A., Pleshakov, D., Rachakonda, T., Chau, A. Q., Weymann, K. B., & Lim, M. M. (2020). Posttraumatic stress disorder increases the odds of REM sleep behavior disorder and other parasomnias in Veterans with and without comorbid traumatic brain injury. *Sleep, 43*(3), zsz237. https://doi.org/10.1093/sleep/zsz237

Ellis, D., & Stuckless, N. (2006). Separation, domestic violence, and divorce mediation. *Conflict Resolution Quarterly, 23*(4), 461–485. https://doi.org/10.1002/crq.150

Elnour, A. A., & Harrison, J. (2008). Lethality of suicide methods. *Injury Prevention, 14*(1), 39–45. https://doi.org/10.1136/ip.2007.016246

Foa, E. B., Bredemeier, K., Acierno, R., Rosenfield, D., Muzzy, W., Tuerk, P. W., Zandberg, L. J., Hart, S., Young-McCaughan, S., Peterson, A. L., & McLean, C. P. (2022). The efficacy of 90-min versus 60-min sessions of prolonged exposure for PTSD: A randomized controlled trial in active-duty military personnel. *Journal of Consulting and Clinical Psychology, 90*(6), 503–512. https://doi.org/10.1037/ccp0000739

Foa, E. B., Chrestman, K. R., & Gilboa-Schechtman, E. (2009). *Prolonged exposure therapy for adolescents with PTSD: Emotional processing of traumatic experiences: Therapist guide.* Oxford University Press.

Foa, E. B., Ehlers, A., Clark, D. M., Tolin, D. F., & Orsillo, S. M. (1999). The Posttraumatic Cognitions Inventory (PTCI): Development and validation. *Psychological Assessment, 11*(3), 303–314. https://doi.org/10.1037/1040-3590.11.3.303

Foa, E. B., Hembree, E. A., Cahill, S. P., Rauch, S. A. M., Riggs, D. S., Feeny, N. C., & Yadin, E. (2005). Randomized trial of prolonged exposure for posttraumatic stress disorder with and without cognitive restructuring: Outcome at academic and community clinics. *Journal of Consulting and Clinical Psychology, 73*(5), 953–964. https://doi.org/10.1037/0022-006X.73.5.953

Foa, E. B., Hembree, E. A., & Rothbaum, B. O. (2007). *Prolonged exposure therapy for PTSD: Emotional processing of traumatic experiences.* Oxford University Press.

Foa, E. B., Hembree, E. A., Rothbaum, B. O., & Rauch, S. A. M. (2019). *Prolonged exposure therapy for PTSD: Emotional processing of traumatic experiences: Therapist guide* (2nd ed.). Oxford University Press. https://doi.org/10.1093/med-psych/9780190926939.001.0001

Foa, E. B., & Kozak, M. J. (1986). Emotional processing of fear: Exposure to corrective information. *Psychological Bulletin, 99*(1), 20–35. https://doi.org/10.1037/0033-2909.99.1.20

Foa, E. B., McLean, C. P., Zang, Y., Zhong, J., Powers, M. B., Kauffman, B. Y., Rauch, S., Porter, K., & Knowles, K. (2016). Psychometric properties of the Posttraumatic Diagnostic Scale for DSM-5 (PDS-5). *Psychological Assessment, 28*(10), 1166–1171. https://doi.org/10.1037/pas0000258

Foa, E. B., McLean, C. P., Zang, Y., Zhong, J., Rauch, S., Porter, K., Knowles, K., Powers, M. B., & Kauffman, B. Y. (2016). Psychometric properties of the Posttraumatic Stress Disorder Symptom Scale Interview for DSM-5 (PSSI-5). *Psychological Assessment, 28*(10), 1159–1165. https://doi.org/10.1037/pas0000259

Foa, E. B., Zinbarg, R., & Rothbaum, B. O. (1992). Uncontrollability and unpredictability in post-traumatic stress disorder: An animal model. *Psychological Bulletin, 112*(2), 218–238. https://doi.org/10.1037/0033-2909.112.2.218

Forbes, C. N., Tull, M. T., Xie, H., Christ, N. M., Brickman, K., Mattin, M., & Wang, X. (2020). Emotional avoidance and social support interact to predict depression symptom severity one year after traumatic exposure. *Psychiatry Research, 284*, 112746. https://doi.org/10.1016/j.psychres.2020.112746

Ford, J. D., & Courtois, C. A. (2021). Complex PTSD and borderline personality disorder. *Borderline Personality Disorder and Emotion Dysregulation, 8*(1), 16. https://doi.org/10.1186/s40479-021-00155-9

Fox, K. R., Harris, J. A., Wang, S. B., Millner, A. J., Deming, C. A., & Nock, M. K. (2020). Self-Injurious Thoughts and Behaviors Interview-Revised: Development, reliability, and validity. *Psychological Assessment, 32*(7), 677–689. https://doi.org/10.1037/pas0000819

Gallagher, M. W. (2017). The Unified Protocol for Posttraumatic Stress Disorder. In D. H. Barlow & T. Farchione (Eds.), *Applications of the Unified Protocol for Transdiagnostic Treatment of Emotional Disorders* (pp. 111–126). Oxford University Press. https://doi.org/10.1093/med-psych/9780190255541.003.0007

Garcia-Moreno, C., Jansen, H. A., Ellsberg, M., Heise, L., & Watts, C. H. (2006). Prevalence of intimate partner violence: Findings from the WHO multi-country study on women's health and domestic violence. *The Lancet, 368*(9543), 1260–1269. https://doi.org/10.1016/S0140-6736(06)69523-8

Gibbs, L. M., Dombrovski, A. Y., Morse, J., Siegle, G. J., Houck, P. R., & Szanto, K. (2009). When the solution is part of the problem: Problem solving in elderly suicide attempters. *International Journal of Geriatric Psychiatry, 24*(12), 1396–1404. https://doi.org/10.1002/gps.2276

Gradus, J. L., Qin, P., Lincoln, A. K., Miller, M., Lawler, E., Sørensen, H. T., & Lash, T. L. (2010). Posttraumatic stress disorder and completed suicide. *American Journal of Epidemiology, 171*(6), 721–727. https://doi.org/10.1093/aje/kwp456

Hammack, S. E., Cooper, M. A., & Lezak, K. R. (2012). Overlapping neurobiology of learned helplessness and conditioned defeat: Implications for PTSD and mood disorders. *Neuropharmacology, 62*(2), 565–575. https://doi.org/10.1016/j.neuropharm.2011.02.024

Harned, M. S., Korslund, K. E., Foa, E. B., & Linehan, M. M. (2012). Treating PTSD in suicidal and self-injuring women with borderline personality disorder: Development and preliminary evaluation of a Dialectical Behavior Therapy Prolonged Exposure Protocol. *Behaviour Research and Therapy, 50*(6), 381–386. https://doi.org/10.1016/j.brat.2012.02.011

Harned, M. S., Korslund, K. E., & Linehan, M. M. (2014). A pilot randomized controlled trial of dialectical behavior therapy with and without the Dialectical Behavior Therapy Prolonged Exposure Protocol for suicidal and self-injuring women with borderline personality disorder and PTSD. *Behaviour Research and Therapy, 55*, 7–17. https://doi.org/10.1016/j.brat.2014.01.008

Harvey, L. J., White, F. A., Hunt, C., & Abbott, M. (2023). Investigating the efficacy of a dialectical behaviour therapy-based universal intervention on adolescent social and emotional well-being outcomes. *Behaviour Research and Therapy, 169*, 104408. https://doi.org/10.1016/j.brat.2023.104408

Hawn, S. E., Cusack, S. E., & Amstadter, A. B. (2020). A systematic review of the self-medication hypothesis in the context of posttraumatic stress disorder and comorbid problematic alcohol use. *Journal of Traumatic Stress, 33*(5), 699–708. https://doi.org/10.1002/jts.22521

Hayes, S. C., Strosahl, K. D., & Wilson, K. G. (1999). *Acceptance and commitment therapy: An experiential approach to behavior change*. Guilford.

Herzog, J. I., Niedtfeld, I., Rausch, S., Thome, J., Mueller-Engelmann, M., Steil, R., Priebe, K., Bohus, M., & Schmahl, C. (2019). Increased recruitment of cognitive control in the presence of traumatic stimuli in complex PTSD. *European Archives of Psychiatry and Clinical Neuroscience, 269*(2), 147–159. https://doi.org/10.1007/s00406-017-0822-x

Houghton, D. C., Spratt, H. M., Keyser-Marcus, L., Bjork, J. M., Neigh, G. N., Cunningham, K. A., Ramey, T., & Moeller, F. G. (2023). Behavioral and neurocognitive factors distinguishing post-traumatic stress comorbidity in substance use disorders. *Translational Psychiatry, 13*(1), 1–11. https://doi.org/10.1038/s41398-023-02591-3

Joiner, T. (2005). *Why people die by suicide*. Harvard University Press.

Jones, L., Hughes, M., & Unterstaller, U. (2001). Post-traumatic stress disorder (PTSD) in victims of domestic violence. *Trauma, Violence & Abuse, 2*(2), 99–195. https://doi.org/10.1177/1524838001002002001

Kanter, J. W., Manos, R. C., Bowe, W. M., Baruch, D. E., Busch, A. M., & Rusch, L. C. (2010). What is behavioral activation? A review of the empirical literature. *Clinical Psychology Review, 30*(6), 608–620. https://doi.org/10.1016/j.cpr.2010.04.001

Kessler, R. C., Aguilar-Gaxiola, S., Alonso, J., Benjet, C., Bromet, E. J., Cardoso, G., Degenhardt, L., de Girolamo, G., Dinolova, R. V., Ferry, F., Florescu, S., Gureje, O., Haro, J. M., Huang, Y., Karam, E. G., Kawakami, N., Lee, S., Lepine, J.-P., Levinson, D., . . . Koenen, K. C. (2017). Trauma and PTSD in the WHO World Mental Health Surveys. *European Journal of Psychotraumatology, 8*(sup5), 1353383. https://doi.org/10.1080/20008198.2017.1353383

Kilpatrick, D. G., Resnick, H. S., Milanak, M. E., Miller, M. W., Keyes, K. M., & Friedman, M. J. (2013). National estimates of exposure to traumatic events and PTSD prevalence using DSM-IV and DSM-5 criteria. *Journal of Traumatic Stress, 26*(5), 537–547. https://doi.org/10.1002/jts.21848

Kind, S., & Otis, J. D. (2019). The interaction between chronic pain and PTSD. *Current Pain and Headache Reports, 23*(12), 91. https://doi.org/10.1007/s11916-019-0828-3

Kircanski, K., Mortazavi, A., Castriotta, N., Baker, A. S., Mystkowski, J. L., Yi, R., & Craske, M. G. (2012). Challenges to the traditional exposure paradigm: Variability in exposure therapy for contamination fears. *Journal of Behavior Therapy and Experimental Psychiatry, 43*(2), 745–751. https://doi.org/10.1016/j.jbtep.2011.10.010

Klonsky, E. D., & May, A. M. (2015). The Three-Step Theory (3ST): A new theory of suicide rooted in the "ideation-to-action" framework. *International Journal of Cognitive Therapy, 8*(2). https://doi.org/10.1521/ijct.2015.8.2.114

Kolbe, V., & Büttner, A. (2020). Domestic violence against men—Prevalence and risk factors. *Deutsches Ärzteblatt International, 117*(31–32), 534–541. https://doi.org/10.3238/arztebl.2020.0534

Kratovic, L., Smith, L. J., & Vujanovic, A. A. (2021). PTSD symptoms, suicidal ideation, and suicide risk in university students: The role of distress tolerance. *Journal of Aggression, Maltreatment & Trauma, 30*(1), 82–100. https://doi.org/10.1080/10926771.2019.1709594

Krause, E. D., Kaltman, S., Goodman, L. A., & Dutton, M. A. (2008). Avoidant coping and PTSD symptoms related to domestic violence exposure: A longitudinal study. *Journal of Traumatic Stress, 21*(1), 83–90. https://doi.org/10.1002/jts.20288

Kroenke, K., Spitzer, R. L., & Williams, J. B. W. (2003). The Patient Health Questionnaire-2: Validity of a two-item depression screener. *Medical Care, 41*(11), 1284–1292. https://doi.org/10.1097/01.MLR.0000093487.78664.3C

Krysinska, K., & Lester, D. (2010). Post-traumatic stress disorder and suicide risk: A systematic review. *Archives of Suicide Research, 14*(1), 1–23. https://doi.org/10.1080/13811110903478997

Kubany, E. S., & Ralston, T. C. (2006). Cognitive therapy for trauma-related guilt and shame. In *Cognitive-behavioral therapies for trauma* (2nd ed., pp. 258–289). Guilford.

LeBouthillier, D. M., McMillan, K. A., Thibodeau, M. A., & Asmundson, G. J. G. (2015). Types and number of traumas associated with suicidal ideation and suicide attempts in PTSD: Findings from a U.S. nationally representative sample. *Journal of Traumatic Stress, 28*(3), 183–190. https://doi.org/10.1002/jts.22010

Lee, K., Noda, Y., Nakano, Y., Ogawa, S., Kinoshita, Y., Funayama, T., & Furukawa, T. A. (2006). Interoceptive hypersensitivity and interoceptive exposure in patients with panic disorder: Specificity and effectiveness. *BMC Psychiatry, 6*(1), 32. https://doi.org/10.1186/1471-244X-6-32

Linehan, M. M. (1993). *Cognitive-behavioral treatment of borderline personality disorder*. Guilford.

Linehan, M. M., Korslund, K. E., Harned, M. S., Gallop, R. J., Lungu, A., Neacsiu, A. D., McDavid, J., Comtois, K. A., & Murray-Gregory, A. M. (2015). Dialectical behavior therapy for high suicide risk in individuals with borderline personality disorder: A randomized clinical trial and component analysis. *JAMA Psychiatry, 72*(5), 475–482. https://doi.org/10.1001/jamapsychiatry.2014.3039

Litz, B. T., & Keane, T. M. (1989). Information processing in anxiety disorders: Application to the understanding of post-traumatic stress disorder. *Clinical Psychology Review, 9*(2), 243–257. https://doi.org/10.1016/0272-7358(89)90030-5

Liverant, G. I., Suvak, M. K., Pineles, S. L., & Resick, P. A. (2012). Changes in posttraumatic stress disorder and depressive symptoms during cognitive processing therapy: Evidence for concurrent change. *Journal of Consulting and Clinical Psychology, 80*(6), 957–967. https://doi.org/10.1037/a0030485

Marx, B. P., & Sloan, D. M. (2005). Peritraumatic dissociation and experiential avoidance as predictors of posttraumatic stress symptomatology. *Behaviour Research and Therapy, 43*(5), 569–583. https://doi.org/10.1016/j.brat.2004.04.004

McCauley, E., Berk, M. S., Asarnow, J. R., Adrian, M., Cohen, J., Korslund, K., Avina, C., Hughes, J., Harned, M., Gallop, R., & Linehan, M. M. (2018). Efficacy of dialectical behavior therapy for adolescents at high risk for suicide: A randomized clinical trial. *JAMA Psychiatry, 75*(8), 777–785. https://doi.org/10.1001/jamapsychiatry.2018.1109

McLean, C. P., Zandberg, L., Brown, L., Zang, Y., Benhamou, K., Dondanville, K. A., Yarvis, J. S., Litz, B. T., Mintz, J., Young-McCaughan, S., Peterson, A. L., & Foa, E. B. for the Consortium for the STRONG STAR Consortium. (2019). Guilt in the treatment of posttraumatic stress disorder among active duty military personnel. *Journal of Traumatic Stress, 32*(4), 616–624. https://doi.org/10.1002/jts.22416

Meiser-Stedman, R., McKinnon, A., Dixon, C., Boyle, A., Smith, P., & Dalgleish, T. (2019). A core role for cognitive processes in the acute onset and maintenance of post-traumatic stress in children and adolescents. *Journal of Child Psychology and Psychiatry, 60*(8), 875–884. https://doi.org/10.1111/jcpp.13054

Meuret, A. E., Rosenfield, D., Wilhelm, F. H., Zhou, E., Conrad, A., Ritz, T., & Roth, W. T. (2011). Do unexpected panic attacks occur spontaneously? *Biological Psychiatry, 70*(10), 985–991. https://doi.org/10.1016/j.biopsych.2011.05.027

Minor, T. R., Plumb, T. N., Schell, C. J., & Pham, A. K. (2011). Brain adenosine signaling in psychological trauma and comorbid depression. In *Neurobiology of post-traumatic stress disorder* (pp. 229–257). Nova Biomedical Books. https://doi.org/10.1007/978-1-4899-1034-9_4

Na, P. J., Yaramala, S. R., Kim, J. A., Kim, H., Goes, F. S., Zandi, P. P., Voort, J. L. V., Sutor, B., Croarkin, P., & Bobo, W. V. (2018). The PHQ-9 Item 9-based screening for suicide risk: A validation study of the Patient Health Questionnaire (PHQ)–9 Item 9 with the Columbia Suicide Severity Rating Scale (C-SSRS). *Journal of Affective Disorders, 232*, 34–40. https://doi.org/10.1016/j.jad.2018.02.045

Nawijn, L., van Zuiden, M., Frijling, J. L., Koch, S. B. J., Veltman, D. J., & Olff, M. (2015). Reward functioning in PTSD: A systematic review exploring the mechanisms underlying anhedonia. *Neuroscience & Biobehavioral Reviews, 51*, 189–204. https://doi.org/10.1016/j.neubiorev.2015.01.019

Nicholls, T. L., Pritchard, M. M., Reeves, K. A., & Hilterman, E. (2013). Risk assessment in intimate partner violence: A systematic review of contemporary approaches. *Partner Abuse, 4*(1), 76–168. https://doi.org/10.1891/1946-6560.4.1.76

O'Donnell, C. J., Schwartz Longacre, L., Cohen, B. E., Fayad, Z. A., Gillespie, C. F., Liberzon, I., Pathak, G. A., Polimanti, R., Risbrough, V., Ursano, R. J., Vander Heide, R. S., Yancy, C. W., Vaccarino, V., Sopko, G., & Stein, M. B. (2021). Posttraumatic stress disorder and cardiovascular disease: State of the science, knowledge gaps, and research opportunities. *JAMA Cardiology, 6*(10), 1207–1216. https://doi.org/10.1001/jamacardio.2021.2530

Olff, M. (2017). Sex and gender differences in post-traumatic stress disorder: An update. *European Journal of Psychotraumatology, 8*(sup4), 1351204. https://doi.org/10.1080/20008198.2017.1351204

Pacella, M. L., Hruska, B., & Delahanty, D. L. (2013). The physical health consequences of PTSD and PTSD symptoms: A meta-analytic review. *Journal of Anxiety Disorders, 27*(1), 33–46. https://doi.org/10.1016/j.janxdis.2012.08.004

Pietrzak, R. H., Goldstein, R. B., Southwick, S. M., & Grant, B. F. (2011). Prevalence and Axis I comorbidity of full and partial posttraumatic stress disorder in the United States: Results from Wave 2 of the National Epidemiologic Survey on Alcohol and Related Conditions. *Journal of Anxiety Disorders, 25*(3), 456–465. https://doi.org/10.1016/j.janxdis.2010.11.010

Pincus, L. E., Brown, L. A., Capaldi, S., Comeau, C., & Foa, E. B. (2022). Trauma exposure and PTSD in Philadelphia community mental health. *Community Mental Health Journal, 58*(3), 547–552. https://doi.org/10.1007/s10597-021-00853-2

Pineles, S. L., Mostoufi, S. M., Ready, C. B., Street, A. E., Griffin, M. G., & Resick, P. A. (2011). Trauma reactivity, avoidant coping, and PTSD symptoms: A moderating relationship? *Journal of Abnormal Psychology, 120*(1), 240–246. https://doi.org/10.1037/a0022123

Pompili, M., Sher, L., Serafini, G., Forte, A., Innamorati, M., Dominici, G., Lester, D., Amore, M., & Girardi, P. (2013). Posttraumatic stress disorder and suicide risk among veterans: A literature review. *Journal of Nervous and Mental Disease, 201*(9), 802. https://doi.org/10.1097/NMD.0b013e3182a21458

Posner, K., Brown, G. K., Stanley, B., Brent, D. A., Yershova, K. V., Oquendo, M. A., Currier, G. W., Melvin, G. A., Greenhill, L., Shen, S., & Mann, J. J. (2011). The Columbia–Suicide Severity Rating Scale: Initial validity and internal consistency findings from three multisite studies with adolescents and adults. *American Journal of Psychiatry, 168*(12), 1266–1277. https://doi.org/10.1176/appi.ajp.2011.10111704

Powers, M. B., Halpern, J. M., Ferenschak, M. P., Gillihan, S. J., & Foa, E. B. (2010). A meta-analytic review of prolonged exposure for posttraumatic stress disorder. *Clinical Psychology Review, 30*(6), 635–641. https://doi.org/10.1016/j.cpr.2010.04.007

Prins, A., Bovin, M. J., Smolenski, D. J., Marx, B. P., Kimerling, R., Jenkins-Guarnieri, M. A., Kaloupek, D. G., Schnurr, P. P., Kaiser, A. P., Leyva, Y. E., & Tiet, Q. Q. (2016). The Primary Care PTSD Screen for DSM-5 (PC-PTSD-5): Development and evaluation within a veteran primary care sample. *Journal of General Internal Medicine, 31*(10), 1206–1211. https://doi.org/10.1007/s11606-016-3703-5

Punton, G., Dodd, A. L., & McNeill, A. (2022). "You're on the waiting list": An interpretive phenomenological analysis of young adults' experiences of waiting lists within mental health services in the UK. *PLOS One, 17*(3), e0265542. https://doi.org/10.1371/journal.pone.0265542

Rauch, S. A. M., Grunfeld, T. E. E., Yadin, E., Cahill, S. P., Hembree, E., & Foa, E. B. (2009). Changes in reported physical health symptoms and social function with prolonged exposure therapy for chronic posttraumatic stress disorder. *Depression and Anxiety, 26*(8), 732–738. https://doi.org/10.1002/da.20518

Reger, G. M., Bourassa, K. J., Smolenski, D., Buck, B., & Norr, A. M. (2019). Lifetime trauma exposure among those with combat-related PTSD: Psychiatric risk among U.S. military personnel. *Psychiatry Research, 278*, 309–314. https://doi.org/10.1016/j.psychres.2019.06.033

Resick, P. A., Monson, C. M., & Chard, K. M. (2016). *Cognitive processing therapy for PTSD: A comprehensive manual.* Guilford Publications.

Rifkin, L. S., Myerberg, L., Gosch, E. A., Norris, L. A., Crane, M. E., & Kendall, P. C. (2021). How to bend but not break an empirically supported treatment for anxiety in youth. In P. C. Kendall (Ed.), *Flexibility within fidelity: Breathing life into a psychological treatment manual* (pp. 175–232). Oxford University Press. https://doi.org/10.1093/med-psych/9780197552155.003.0011

Roberts, N. P., Back, S. E., Mueser, K. T., & Murray, L. K. (2020). Treatment considerations for PTSD comorbidities. In *Effective treatments for PTSD: Practice guidelines from the International Society for Traumatic Stress Studies* (3rd ed., pp. 417–450). Guilford.

Robinaugh, D. J., Marques, L., Traeger, L. N., Marks, E. H., Sung, S. C., Gayle Beck, J., Pollack, M. H., & Simon, N. M. (2011). Understanding the relationship of perceived social support to post-trauma cognitions and posttraumatic stress disorder. *Journal of Anxiety Disorders, 25*(8), 1072–1078. https://doi.org/10.1016/j.janxdis.2011.07.004

Roddy, J., & Dubrow-Marshall, R. (2023). Understanding domestic abuse. In *Working with Client Experiences of Domestic Abuse* (pp. 22–42). Routledge. https://doi.org/10.4324/9781003253266-3

Rosen, V., & Ayers, G. (2020). An update on the complexity and importance of accurately diagnosing post-traumatic stress disorder and comorbid traumatic brain injury. *Neuroscience Insights, 15*, 2633105520907895. https://doi.org/10.1177/2633105520907895

Rosenbaum, S., Stubbs, B., Ward, P. B., Steel, Z., Lederman, O., & Vancampfort, D. (2015). The prevalence and risk of metabolic syndrome and its components among people with posttraumatic stress disorder: A systematic review and meta-analysis. *Metabolism, 64*(8), 926–933. https://doi.org/10.1016/j.metabol.2015.04.009

Ross, M. E., Vidair, H. B., & Fordsham, N. (2022). *Do psychologists accept, prefer, and use imaginal exposure over other techniques to treat generalized anxiety? A survey.* SSRN Scholarly Paper 4035457. https://doi.org/10.2139/ssrn.4035457

Roth-Rawald, J., Maaß, U., Mai, S., & Weck, F. (2023). Exposure therapy for health anxiety: Effectiveness and response rates in routine care of an outpatient clinic. *Journal of Clinical Psychology, 79*(12), 2884–2898. https://doi.org/10.1002/jclp.23587

Rudd, M. D. (2006). Fluid vulnerability theory: A cognitive approach to understanding the process of acute and chronic suicide risk. In *Cognition and suicide: Theory, research, and therapy* (pp. 355–368). American Psychological Association. https://doi.org/10.1037/11377-016

Ruglass, L. M., Morgan-López, A. A., Saavedra, L. M., Hien, D. A., Fitzpatrick, S., Killeen, T. K., Back, S. E., & López-Castro, T. (2020). Measurement nonequivalence of the Clinician-Administered PTSD Scale by race/ethnicity: Implications for quantifying posttraumatic stress disorder severity. *Psychological Assessment, 32*(11), 1015–1027. https://doi.org/10.1037/pas0000943

Rytwinski, N. K., Scur, M. D., Feeny, N. C., & Youngstrom, E. A. (2013). The co-occurrence of major depressive disorder among individuals with posttraumatic stress disorder: A meta-analysis. *Journal of Traumatic Stress, 26*(3), 299–309. https://doi.org/10.1002/jts.21814

Scharff, A., Ortiz, S. N., Forrest, L. N., & Smith, A. R. (2021). Comparing the clinical presentation of eating disorder patients with and without trauma history and/or comorbid PTSD. *Eating Disorders, 29*(1), 88–102. https://doi.org/10.1080/10640266.2019.1642035

Schnurr, P. P., Friedman, M. J., Foy, D. W., Shea, M. T., Hsieh, F. Y., Lavori, P. W., Glynn, S. M., Wattenberg, M., & Bernardy, N. C. (2003). Randomized trial of trauma-focused group therapy for posttraumatic stress disorder: Results from a Department of Veterans Affairs cooperative study. *Archives of General Psychiatry, 60*(5), 481–489. https://doi.org/10.1001/archpsyc.60.5.481

Schnurr, P. P., Lunney, C. A., & Sengupta, A. (2004). Risk factors for the development versus maintenance of posttraumatic stress disorder. *Journal of Traumatic Stress, 17*(2), 85–95. https://doi.org/10.1023/B:JOTS.0000022614.21794.f4

Schuettler, D., & Boals, A. (2011). The path to posttraumatic growth versus posttraumatic stress disorder: Contributions of event centrality and coping. *Journal of Loss and Trauma, 16*(2), 180–194. https://doi.org/10.1080/15325024.2010.519273

Seligman, M. E. P. (1972). Learned helplessness. *Annual Review of Medicine, 23*, 407–412. https://doi.org/10.1146/annurev.me.23.020172.002203

Sheynin, J., Shind, C., Radell, M., Ebanks-Williams, Y., Gilbertson, M. W., Beck, K. D., & Myers, C. E. (2017). Greater avoidance behavior in individuals with posttraumatic stress disorder symptoms. *Stress, 20*(3), 285–293. https://doi.org/10.1080/10253890.2017.1309523

Simon, N., Roberts, N. P., Lewis, C. E., van Gelderen, M. J., & Bisson, J. I. (2019). Associations between perceived social support, posttraumatic stress disorder (PTSD) and complex PTSD (CPTSD): Implications for treatment. *European Journal of Psychotraumatology, 10*(1). https://doi.org/10.1080/20008198.2019.1573129

Sloan, D. M., & Marx, B. P. (2019). *Written exposure therapy for PTSD*. American Psychological Press. https://www.apa.org/pubs/books/4317524

Stanley, B., Brown, G. K., Brenner, L. A., Galfalvy, H. C., Currier, G. W., Knox, K. L., Chaudhury, S. R., Bush, A. L., & Green, K. L. (2018). Comparison of the Safety Planning Intervention with follow-up vs usual care of suicidal patients treated in the emergency department. *JAMA Psychiatry, 75*(9), 894–900. https://doi.org/10.1001/jamapsychiatry.2018.1776

Stanley, I. H., Boffa, J. W., & Joiner, T. E. (2019). PTSD from a suicide attempt: Phenomenological and diagnostic considerations. *Psychiatry, 82*(1), 57–71. https://doi.org/10.1080/00332747.2018.1485373

Stanley, I. H., Hom, M. A., Boffa, J. W., Stage, D. L., & Joiner, T. E. (2019). PTSD from a suicide attempt: An empirical investigation among suicide attempt survivors. *Journal of Clinical Psychology, 75*(10), 1879–1895. https://doi.org/10.1002/jclp.22833

Stevens, D., Wilcox, H. C., MacKinnon, D. F., Mondimore, F. M., Schweizer, B., Jancic, D., Coryell, W. H., Weissman, M. M., Levinson, D. F., & Potash, J. B. (2013). Posttraumatic stress disorder increases risk for suicide attempt in adults with recurrent major depression. *Depression and Anxiety, 30*(10), 940–946. https://doi.org/10.1002/da.22160

Stone, D. M. (2018). *Vital Signs:* Trends in state suicide rates – United States, 1999–2016 and circumstances contributing to suicide – 27 states, 2015. *MMWR. Morbidity and Mortality Weekly Report, 67*. https://doi.org/10.15585/mmwr.mm6722a1

Swart, S., Wildschut, M., Draijer, N., Langeland, W., & Smit, J. H. (2020). Dissociative subtype of posttraumatic stress disorder or PTSD with comorbid dissociative disorders: Comparative evaluation of clinical profiles. *Psychological Trauma: Theory, Research, Practice, and Policy, 12*(1), 38–45. https://doi.org/10.1037/tra0000474

Tarrier, N., & Gregg, L. (2004). Suicide risk in civilian PTSD patients. *Social Psychiatry and Psychiatric Epidemiology, 39*(8), 655–661. https://doi.org/10.1007/s00127-004-0799-4

Tuerk, P. W., Wangelin, B., Rauch, S. A. M., Dismuke, C. E., Yoder, M., Myrick, H., Eftekhari, A., & Acierno, R. (2013). Health service utilization before and after evidence-based treatment for PTSD. *Psychological Services, 10*(4), 401–409. https://doi.org/10.1037/a0030549

Utzon-Frank, N., Breinegaard, N., Bertelsen, M., Borritz, M., Eller, N. H., Nordentott, M., Olesen, K., Rod, N. H., Rugulies, R., & Bonde, J. P. (2014). Occurrence of delayed-onset post-traumatic stress disorder: A systematic review and meta-analysis of prospective studies. *Scandinavian Journal of Work, Environment & Health, 40*(3), 215–229. https://doi.org/10.5271/sjweh.3420

van Marle, H. (2015). PTSD as a memory disorder. *European Journal of Psychotraumatology, 6*(1), 27633. https://doi.org/10.3402/ejpt.v6.27633

van Minnen, A., Harned, M. S., Zoellner, L., & Mills, K. (2012). Examining potential contraindications for prolonged exposure therapy for PTSD. *European Journal of Psychotraumatology, 3*(1), 18805. https://doi.org/10.3402/ejpt.v3i0.18805

van Minnen, A., Zoellner, L. A., Harned, M. S., & Mills, K. (2015). Changes in comorbid conditions after prolonged exposure for PTSD: A literature review. *Current Psychiatry Reports, 17*(3), 17. https://doi.org/10.1007/s11920-015-0549-1

Weathers, F. W., Bovin, M. J., Lee, D. J., Sloan, D. M., Schnurr, P. P., Kaloupek, D. G., Keane, T. M., & Marx, B. P. (2018). The Clinician-Administered PTSD Scale for DSM-5 (CAPS-5): Development and initial psychometric evaluation in military veterans. *Psychological Assessment, 30*(3), 383–395. https://doi.org/10.1037/pas0000486

Weaver, S. S., Kroska, E. B., Ross, M. C., Sartin-Tarm, A., Sellnow, K. A., Schaumberg, K., Kiehl, K. A., Koenigs, M., & Cisler, J. M. (2020). Sacrificing reward to avoid threat: Characterizing PTSD in the context of a trauma-related approach-avoidance conflict task. *Journal of Abnormal Psychology, 129*(5), 457–468. https://doi.org/10.1037/abn0000528

Weiss, T., Skelton, K., Phifer, J., Jovanovic, T., Gillespie, C. F., Smith, A., Umpierrez, G., Bradley, B., & Ressler, K. J. (2011). Posttraumatic stress disorder is a risk factor for metabolic syndrome in an impoverished urban population. *General Hospital Psychiatry, 33*(2), 135–142. https://doi.org/10.1016/j.genhosppsych.2011.01.002

Wells, S. Y., Morland, L. A., Torres, E. M., Kloezeman, K., Mackintosh, M.-A., & Aarons, G. A. (2019). The development of a brief version of the Posttraumatic Cognitions Inventory (PTCI-9). *Assessment, 26*(2), 193–208. https://doi.org/10.1177/1073191116685401

White, S. J., Sin, J., Sweeney, A., Salisbury, T., Wahlich, C., Montesinos Guevara, C. M., Gillard, S., Brett, E., Allwright, L., Iqbal, N., Khan, A., Perot, C., Marks, J., & Mantovani, N. (2024). Global prevalence and mental health outcomes of intimate partner violence among women: A systematic review and meta-analysis. *Trauma, Violence & Abuse, 25*(1), 494–511. https://doi.org/10.1177/15248380231155529

White, W. F., Burgess, A., Dalgleish, T., Halligan, S., Hiller, R., Oxley, A., Smith, P., & Meiser-Stedman, R. (2022). Prevalence of the dissociative subtype of post-traumatic stress disorder: A systematic review and meta-analysis. *Psychological Medicine, 52*(9), 1629–1644. https://doi.org/10.1017/S0033291722001647

Whiteside, S. P. H. (2023). Examining community clinicians use of imaginal exposure with childhood anxiety disorders. *Child Psychiatry & Human Development*. https://doi.org/10.1007/s10578-023-01556-3

Williams, J. M. G., Barnhofer, T., Crane, C., & Beck, A. T. (2005). Problem solving deteriorates following mood challenge in formerly depressed patients with a history of suicidal ideation. *Journal of Abnormal Psychology, 114*(3), 421–431. https://doi.org/10.1037/0021-843X.114.3.421

Yip, P. S., Caine, E., Yousuf, S., Chang, S.-S., Wu, K. C.-C., & Chen, Y.-Y. (2012). Means restriction for suicide prevention. *The Lancet, 379*(9834), 2393–2399. https://doi.org/10.1016/S0140-6736(12)60521-2

Zhu, Y., Rodebaugh, T., Narine, K., & Brown, L. A. (2022). Idiographic dynamics between suicide ideation and depression, anxiety and posttraumatic stress symptoms in persons living with HIV: A pilot study. *Journal for Person-Oriented Research, 8*(2), 71–86. https://doi.org/10.17505/jpor.2022.24856

Appendix: Resources and Tools

The following materials for your book can be downloaded free of charge once you register on the Hogrefe website.

Handout 1: Rationale for CBT for PTSD
Handout 2: Common Questions and Answers for Patients Embarking on Exposure Therapy
Handout 3: Brainstorming *in Vivo* Exposure Ideas
Handout 4: Brainstorming Interoceptive Exposure Ideas

How to proceed:

DOWNLOAD

1. Go to www.hgf.io/media and create a user account. If you already have one, please log in.

2. Go to **My supplementary materials** in your account dashboard and enter the code below. You will automatically be redirected to the download area, where you can access and download the supplementary materials.

   Code: B-99A3N8

To make sure you have permanent direct access to all the materials, we recommend that you download them and save them on your computer.

Handout 1

Rationale for CBT for PTSD

- Cognitive behavioral therapy (CBT) is a very effective treatment for posttraumatic stress disorder (PTSD)
- In CBT, we focus on understanding **three parts of an emotion**: (1) thoughts; (2) behaviors; (3) physical sensations.
- These three components **affect each other**. That means that how a person thinks about a situation affects how they are tempted to behave in the situation, which also affects how their body feels in that situation.
- You and your therapist will work on different **skills** to directly address each of these three components.
- Patients with PTSD often notice that they are very tempted to **avoid thinking about the trauma** or doing things that remind them of the trauma. Sometimes this makes it such that their lives become increasingly narrow. This is very understandable but also unfulfilling. In CBT for PTSD, you and your therapist will work together to gradually practice **growing your life in the direction that matters to you.** The therapist will help you with this with a behavioral strategy called **exposure practice.** One type of exposure practice is for addressing painful memories, another is for addressing situations that are avoided and a third is for addressing bodily sensations that are uncomfortable.
- You and your therapist will also work together to understand **negative trauma-related thoughts** about yourself, other people, or the world that affect your PTSD symptoms.
- Depending on your symptoms, you and your therapist might also use some strategies to help tackle depression. In this context, you and your therapist will use behavioral activation to help you **build your self-confidence and empowerment.**
- At all times in treatment, **you are in control.** Your therapist will serve in the role of a coach who is an expert in PTSD. Your therapist will never pressure you into doing things that you aren't ready to do. They are here to give you opportunities to move your life in a positive direction.

This is a **preview** of the content that is available in the downloadable material of this book. Please see p. 163 for instructions on how to obtain the full-sized, printable PDF.

Handout 2

Common Questions and Answers for Patients Embarking on Exposure Therapy

What is exposure therapy?

Exposure therapy involves approaching situations, memories, or sensations that you would otherwise prefer to avoid. In the short run, avoidance might give you some relief from anxiety and distress. In the long run, avoidance makes anxiety and distress worse. Exposure therapy breaks the cycle of avoidance.

What kinds of exposures will I do?

You and your therapist will make collaborative decisions about what kinds of exposures might be most helpful to you. This might include exposure to safe situations that make you anxious, to talking about difficult memories of the past, or to uncomfortable physical sensations.

How will I do exposures?

First, you and your therapist will discuss what you need to learn about your anxiety. This is different for everyone. Next, you and your therapist will decide on a manageable first exposure to practice. Then, you will do the exposure and report back about how it went. Finally, you and your therapist will decide what kinds of exposures would be most helpful as a next step.

Isn't it dangerous to make myself feel stressed out?

Research shows that for most people, stress itself is not dangerous. Stress tends to lead to bad outcomes because of the changes that people make to their lives that are unhealthy. When stress is interpreted as a challenge to be overcome, and when people have the support to overcome stress, there is nothing dangerous about stress alone. If you're worried, you can always talk to your physician about what is and is not safe for you. Also, most people find that once they get in the habit of doing exposures, stress is actually reduced and they feel more capable of handling stressful situations in the future.

What if I'm scared to do exposures?

If there is an exposure that makes you feel a bit nervous, that probably means that you are on the right track. If the activity were totally relaxing, it would not even count as an exposure. Don't push yourself too far too soon but remember that most people feel nervous about exposures. That's usually a sign that the activity is important to you in some way! Consider discussing your concerns with your therapist for support. Anxiety about exposures is completely normal and healthy.

Handout 3

Brainstorming *in Vivo* Exposure Ideas

Let's brainstorm some options for *in vivo* exposure practice. Remember, just because you write it on this sheet does not mean that you are committing to doing it. This is just about getting possibilities on paper.

What **places** do you avoid since the trauma?

___

___

- Note whether certain details would alter your comfort level with those places, like time of day or how busy the place is: ___

Who are **people** that you avoid since the trauma?

___

___

What **objects** do you avoid since the trauma?

___

___

What **situations** do you avoid since the trauma?

___

___

What **activities** do you avoid since the trauma??

___

___

Prepping for *in Vivo* Exposure

For any of the places, people, objects, situations, or activities that you avoid listed above, work with your therapist to choose one on which to focus. Write it down here:

___

This is a **preview** of the content that is available in the downloadable material of this book. Please see p. 163 for instructions on how to obtain the full-sized, printable PDF.

In vivo exposure practice (describe):

Hypothesis: In the worst-case scenario, what do you predict might happen if you do this exposure?

What kinds of safety behaviors do you want to reduce during the exposure?

What do you need to tell yourself to stick with the situation, even if it is anxiety provoking?

Processing the *in Vivo* Exposure

What did you notice during the *in vivo* exposure? Did the worst-case scenario that you wrote above happen?

What is your takeaway from the *in vivo* exposure?

What do you need to learn next?

Handout 4

Brainstorming Interoceptive Exposure Ideas

Let's brainstorm some options for interoceptive exposure practice. Remember, just because you write it on this sheet does not mean that you are committing to doing it. This is just about getting possibilities on paper.

What are some **physical sensations** that you avoid in general?

____

____

What **activities** do you avoid because they may bring on uncomfortable physical sensations?

____

____

What **food, beverage, or medications** do you avoid because they may bring on uncomfortable sensations?

____

____

What **clothes** do you avoid wearing because they may bring on uncomfortable sensations?

____

____

What **situations** do you avoid because they may bring on uncomfortable sensations?

____

____

Prepping for Interoceptive Exposure

For any of the uncomfortable sensations (or situations that provoke uncomfortable sensations) above, work with your therapist to choose one on which to focus. Write it down here:

____

This is a **preview** of the content that is available in the downloadable material of this book. Please see p. 163 for instructions on how to obtain the full-sized, printable PDF.

Interoceptive exposure practice (describe):

How long should you do this practice? Ideally, select a time that will allow the uncomfortable sensations to intensify:

Hypothesis: In the worst-case scenario, what do you predict might happen if you do this exposure?

What kinds of safety behaviors do you want to reduce during the exposure?

What do you need to tell yourself to stick with the interoceptive exposure, even if it is anxiety provoking?

Processing the Interoceptive Exposure

What did you notice during the interoceptive exposure? Did the worst-case scenario that you wrote above happen?

What is your takeaway from the interoceptive exposure?

What do you need to learn next?

This is a **preview** of the content that is available in the downloadable material of this book. Please see p. 163 for instructions on how to obtain the full-sized, printable PDF.

Peer Commentaries

"This book is a clear and practical guide for mental health providers at any stage of their career seeking to personalize and optimize CBT for trauma survivors. Drawing on research data, established interventions, and clinical experiences, it offers rich illustrations and hands-on tools for real-world practice. It is very comprehensive, yet accessible, and addresses key factors in providing CBT optimally to trauma survivors, including therapeutic strategies, barriers to engagement with and effective implementation of CBT, contextual influences for the client, and training/supervision."

Ateka A. Contractor, PhD, Professor, Department of Psychology, University of North Texas, Denton, TX

"Dr Lily Brown provides a concise and yet comprehensive overview of CBT for PTSD in practice. Both experienced providers and those new to CBT for PTSD will find useful tips and specific tools to help them in their work with patients, training other providers, and consideration for program development. She provides clear background for her recommendations based on experimental psychopathology and clinical trials research. The handouts and figures provide quick guides to complex issues, like what is the role of the therapist in imaginal exposure, how to set up the in vivo *hierarchy, etc. I would recommend this book for anyone clinically working with survivors of trauma."*

Sheila A. M. Rauch, PhD, ABPP, Professor, Emory University School of Medicine, Deputy Director, Emory Healthcare Veterans Program, Atlanta, GA

"This book distills the best of evidence-based trauma-focused psychotherapy for PTSD – like cognitive processing therapy and prolonged exposure – into clear, practical guidance you can use right away. Grounded in science and packed with real-world examples, it's an indispensable companion for both new and seasoned clinicians seeking to elevate their trauma-focused clinical practice."

Lori A. Zoellner, PhD, Professor, Department of Psychology, University of Washington, Director, UW Center for Anxiety and Traumatic Stress, Seattle, WA